Kombrinck's Concise Anesthesi

WARNING

Don't study review books such as this unless …
#1 You have a foundation, ie. previously have read an entire source (Baby Miller, Morgan, etc).
#2 You have no time and there is a test next week.

This was originally created during my residency training as an Anesthesiology one-liner study guide for the ABA/ASA Board exam, Anesthesia Knowledge Test (AKT), and In-Training Exam (ITE).

For Anesthesiology Residents:

The In Training Exam (ITE) is in March of each year & is 4 hrs long, with roughly 225 MCQs: A-type (standard), R-type (hardest), & G-sets (no big deal). That's 64 sec per question. It is broken down into subheadings that this book is based on. If questions about what material is fair game, go to ABA website and ITE content outline & there is a 41 page document that summarizes the expected breadth of your knowledge to score 100th percentile. Good luck with that. If you know this book "luke-warm" turkey, you will get at least 35th percentile (solid pass). The board itself is esoteric, with quite a few disagreements between questions, studies, books, and the writers. These facts account for the possibility of different formatting, duplications, as well as errors that could be argued either way. There is considerable overlap between titles of chapters, with no easy way to reconcile this. If you don't understand my abbreviations, content, or see errors contact me for 2nd edtion edits or study harder ☺. My email is mckselect@gmail.com.

For All Anesthesia Professionals:

This is a "one-liner" format for dense, high-yield question related content. It is a compilation of my random, although sometimes deliberate, writings throughout my CA1-3 years of residency training. For example, sometimes 3 lines are all related to a prior line. However, I tried to at least alphabetize when possible. The way to use this is to read each line, stop & think on it, conceptualize it, and then move on. Do not just breeze through it. It's very dense in some areas (hence all the abbreviations). I have updated the information as of the first quarter of 2013, which should be test worthy material for the next 10 plus years. It should help on most tests on anesthesia and/or serve as a quick reference to keep in your locker at work. I hope you enjoy and dominate your boards!

- J. Kombrinck, MD

About the Author

I am one of three sibling anesthesia providers and studied undergraduate science and medicine at the University of Florida. I completed residency training in the Deep South at the University of Mississippi Medical Center in Jackson, MS. I am ever grateful for the incredible training experience I received there. I then completed fellowship training at the University of North Carolina Chapel Hill in Regional Anesthesia and Acute Pain Management. I enjoy hands on education of others. However, I am willing to sacrifice and publish this text for the hopeful benefit of those I can't be near.

Dedicated to Moya and Ian. ☺

Table of Contents

1. Equipment, Physics, Monitoring

Equipment

Tanks: O2 full at 625L and 2200psi. Air full at 625L and 1800psi. CO2/N20 840/750, full at 1590L.

N2O tank full at 1590L has 750psi until ¾ empty (~400L). Then pressure begins to fall. Different from others.

O2 flush valve rate is 35-75L/min. It bypasses the low-pressure system risking barotrauma.

Heat of vaporization is amt of calories req at specific temp to convert 1g liquid into vapor.

Variable bypass (modern vaporizors) splits flow into 2 portions, flow over anesthetic & flow bypassing it.

Splitting ratio dependent on agent (saturated vapor pressure), temp, & vapor conc selected.

The more increased the altitude (lower barometric pressure) the greater the vaporizer output.

Measured-flow vaporizors (non-concentration calibrated) include copper kettle and Vernitrol.

Copper kettle is copper to minimize heat loss & provide a measurable temp. What goes in vaporizer comes out.

Semi-closed circle system is most common (UMC). Semi open req high FGF rates. Closed is total rebreathing.

Jackson Rees (MapF) popular in peds, minimal dead space, requires high FGF, lack humidification.

Bain (MapD) has APL next to reservoir. Inner tube can kink (hypoxia). Best for *controlled vent*, need high FGF.

If unidirectional valves are working properly the only dead space in circle system is bt the y-piece & the pt.

The reservoir bag limits pressure in breathing circuit to 60mmHg even if APL is closed.

Fail safe valve (pressure sensitive shutoff valve) is set to 25psi to prevent flow of N2O if O2 doesn't have 25psi.

Bellows that rise during exhalation (ascending) are preferred because will not fill if there is a leak or disconnect.

Descending bellows carry the risk of not alarming when a disconnect has occurred bc can entrain room air.

NIOSH limits contamination of OR atmosphere to < 25ppm N20 & < 0.5ppm of volatile w/N20, <2ppm volatile only.

If excess vaccum is placed on scavenging system, negative pressures can occur in the breathing sytem.

The air in the OR should be exchanged at least 15x/hr by the OR ventilation system.

Size of CO2 canister should be > or equal to the pt's Tidal Volume to prevent rebreathing.

Soda Lime: CO2 absorbent , CaOH (80%), NaOH (4%), KOH (1%), H2O (15%).

Amsorb Plus: CO2 absorbent, CaOH (80%), H20 (15%), CaCl2.

Baralyme (no longer available) when dessicated will cause intense exothermic rxn with Sevo (fire).

Soda lime generates compound A with Sevo & CO with VAs. Amsorb Plus does not do either.

Carbon monoxide produced (Baralyme > Soda lime) in decreasing order: Des/Enf > Iso >> Halo/Sevo

Mixture of CO2 with CaOH is exothermic (Sodalyme and Baralyme).

Most impt preop vent checks are calibration of O2 monior, leak checks of low-pressure & of breathing systems.

Always do leak check of breathing system. Will pass even if unidirectional valves are incompetent/stuck shut.

If cleaning equipment use bleach to disinfect for AIDs patients. Destroys HIV.

The O2 cylinder pressure regulator ↓'s pressure from 2200psig to 45psig. N20 from 745psig to 45psig.

Anesthesia workstation includes ONLY components needed to "administer anesthesia". Not suction, etc.

O2 analyzer best to detect flow meter leak. Always needed to ensure no hypoxic gas mixture.

No ferromagnetic devices in MRI. Titanium, aluminum, copper, silver are OK. Nickel & Cobalt not ok.

If missile injury, turn off magnet; remove patient as magnet will become very cold.

Upper airway obstruction during MRI causes unacceptable motion artifact.

Physics

Laminar fluid/gas flow influenced by viscosity. Helium does not improve, like it does turbulent flow.

Turbulent (orifice) flow influenced by density. When Reynolds # >2000, laminar flow becomes turbulent.

Hagan Pouisielle = laminar flow (velocity) thru tube; $V = [\pi r^4 \Delta P] / 8L\mu$; impt numbers are the 4 & 8.

Hagan Pouisielle also = Resistance = $(8L\mu)/ (\pi r^4)$; μ = viscosity

Reynolds # = dimensionless # that gives ratio of inertial ($\rho V2/L$) forces over viscous ($\mu V/L2$) forces.

Grahams Law: diffusion coefficient inversely proportional to square root of molecular weight.

Frank-Starling = (vol/pressure) is larger preload results in incr'd CO/SV. EF normally remains same.

CO = SV x HR; SVR=(MAP-CVP)/CO x 80; Resistance = pressure / flow.

Think of V=IR (Ohm's) so then R=V/I, so SVR (resistance) = pressure(voltage)/flow(current).

Oncotic/Interstitial pressure equation = $Jv = Kf ([Pc - Pi] - \partial [\pi c - \pi i])$

Fick's Equation: VO2 = CO x (CaO2 – CvO2); calculate VO2 (O2 consumption). Normal is 3.5mL/kg/min

Fick's Diffusion: Gas thru membrane directly prop to pressure, area, & inversely to thickness/molecular wt

Kf is a constant ,Jv is net fluid movement, ∂ is the reflection coefficient.

Compliance = $\Delta V/\Delta P$; Velocity = $\Delta D/\Delta t$; Ultrasound (U/S): Nyquist limit is maximum detectable f shift.

U/S: Power output = electrical energy given to transducer; Gain = amplification of returning signals

U/S: Waves described by f (Hz=1cycle/sec), velocity (m/s), wavlength (mm), & amplitude (dB).

U/S: shorter λ penetrate shorter distances, Image resolution is no greater than 1-2 λ (1mm).

U/S: Velocity (f x λ) of sound thru bone is 3000 m/s & thru soft tissue is 1540 m/s.

U/S: 1Mhz transducer = 30cm depth penetration; 5mHz = 6cm, 20MHz = 1.5cm.

U/S: 6 dB change is doubling or halfing, & 40dB change represents 100x difference.

U/S: Acoustic impedance depends on tissue density (most impt) & propogation velocity of the tissue.

Echo: SV = πr^2 (of AV) x VTI (across AV); Stenotic pressure gradients $\Delta P = 4v^2$

Critical temp is temp above which substance can't be pressurized into a liquid. O2 = -120 degrees, always gas!

If machine calibated at sea level then used in Denver, Vp/Vb ratio ↑ s. Delivered […] is > than indicated.

Monitoring

Req ASA monitors for GETA are sat, EKG, BP q5min, FiO2 monitor, EtCO2, Vent disconnect alarm.

All anesthesia requires monitoring of oxygenation, ventilation, and circulation.

EKG: Lead I looks across chest, Lead II looks along long axis of heart. V5 (need 5 lead) looks at LV.

EKG: intraop most concerned for STΔs & rhythm (lead II best). 3-lead shows only Lead I & II.

EKG: ischemia detected via ST or T wave Δs. Lead V5 is best (75%). Leads II, V4, V5 are 96% sensitive.

ESWL shocks are triggered based on EKG at 20 msec after the R wave = absolute refractory period.

BP cuff width should be 40% circumference of the arm. Too small (falsely high BP read) & visa-versa.

We use dinamap oscillometry which overestimated diastolic by 10mmHg. 1.34 cm H20 = 1 mmHg.

For A-lines keep tranducer at level of center of heart. For every 15cm up or down there is 10mm error Δ BP.

A-line indications: expect wide HDΔs, frequent labs, large fluid shifts, inability to monitor via non-invasive.

CVP: true measured on end expiration (vent off). Nl CVP (-2 – 6cmH20) spont vent & 4-12 (mechanical).

CVP: a (RA contract), c (tricusp bulge), x descent (RV contract), v (RA filling) y descent (RA begins to empty).

CVP: canon A waves when contraction against closed tricusp. In heart block or nodal rhythms.

Pulmonary Art catheter is 110cm plastic tube containing 4 lumens with 1.5mL capacity balloon.

Pulm cath estimates EVEDP indirectly by PAOP (wedge). Nl is 8-18 mmHg. Frank pulm edema at 30.

Nl PvO_2 (MvO_2) is 40mmHg (sat 75%). Lowered by ↓ O2 delivery, ↓ CO, or an ↑ in O2 consumption.

TEE measures wall motion abn, cardiac function, SV, valve fxn, intracardiac air, filling pressures, velocities.

Doppler shift used for velocitities in TEE. Max (in PW) measureable is ½ the pulse rep freq = Nyquist limit.

Use continuous wave Doppler for higher velocities than could be measured by Pulse wave Doppler (PW).

Pulse ox: based on Beers-Lambert Law correlates solute conc (Hb) to intensity of light transmitted thru solution.

Pulse ox: measures the amount of ↑'d absorbance seen in pulsatile component (venous is baseline absorbtion).

Pulse ox: errors due to metHb (sat 85%), COHb (need co-oximetry). IV dyes will lower sats as well.

Pulse ox: most common alert to problem. Blue nail polish affects the sat probe the most (fixed artifactual value).

SSEPs: measure intregrity of dorsal columns (sensory) of the SC. Warn against posterior SC ischemia.

SSEP electrodes stimulate at large nerves (median, post tib) and record on scalp (near spinal cord).

SSEP: NMBDs do NOT affect. VAs ↓ amp & ↑ latency. Etomidate/Ketamine ↑ both.

MEPs uncommon. Stimulate on scalp & record on muscle. Difficult to obtain & prone to inaccuracy.

Capnography: confirms ventilation (after 3 breaths), estimates $PaCO_2$, & evaluates dead space.

Capnography: ↑ $EtCO_2$ = hypovent, MH, sepsis, rebreathing, bicarb given, CO_2 insufflation.

Capnography: ↓ $EtCO_2$ = hypervent, hypothermia, ↓ CO, PE, disconnect, cardiac arrest.

EEG monitoring encompasses spontaneous EEG & electromyographic (EMG) activity (BIS, Narcotrend).

BIS algorhythmically processes EEG into single digit (unitless) number. 45-60 is goal. If >70, ↑ recall.

BIS affected by hypothermia, liver failure, EMG contamination, & other factors (ie head trauma, unknown).

Recall incidence is 1:500. Hearing last to go & 1st to come back. Highest in obstetrics, cardiac, & trauma.

Temp: Anesthesia ↓ thermoregulation, vasodilates. Core body temp ↓ 1-1.5 degrees C in 1st hr after induction.

Temp: Hypothermia delays recovery, causes arrhythmias, & impairs coag times & wound healing.

Temp: Best core is PA cath, then TM probe, then bladder. Rectal, esophageal should be used as trendometer.

Temp: Heat loss: Radiation > Conduction > Convection > Evaporation. Body warmer (bair hugger) best.

VA measured by mono & polychromatic (we use) infrared spectroscopy, mass spec, & Raman spec.

TOF stimulus level is 2Hz. Tetanus is 50-100Hz. Post-tetanic stimulation measured after 5-second tetanus.

Let go current is 20 milliA. Maximal current leak for ICDs is 10 microA. 50 microA -> Vfib.

Line isolation monitor (LIM) continually monitors all potential parallel leakage (impedance) paths to ground.

LIM shows what current could flow to a person (1000 Ohms) if a line conductor (defective equip) is touched.

LIM alarms if faulty piece of equipment is plugged into output sockets of the Isolated Power System.

Low pressure monitor alarm is first to detect circuit disconnect.

2. Math/Equations, Stats, Computers

Math/Equations

Alveolar gas eqn: $PAO2=(Pb - 47)FiO2 - PaCO2/0.8$, relates FiO2 to PAO2. nl PA02 on 100% ~600mmHg.

Alveolar Gas Equation: Calculate via: $Aa = P_A - P_a$; $P_A = 713(FiO2) - PaCO2/0.8$

Bohr Equation (dead space:tidal vol ratio) = $Vd/Vt = (PaCO2 - PETCO2)/PaCO2$, normal is <0.3. Normal V/Q is 0.8

$CO = SV \times HR$; $SVR=(MAP-CVP)/CO \times 80$; Resistance = pressure / flow.

$EF = SV/EDV$ or $(EDV-ESV)/EDV$; $SV = EDV - ESV$

EtCO2 5-10mmHg lower than PaCO2 bc anatomic dead space always present (decr'd physiologic dead space).

$F_ENa = (U_{Na} - P_{Cr}) / (U_{Cr} - P_{Na})$; Water deficit = $0.6 \times kg \times [1-(140/Na)]$

Fick Equation: $VO2 = CO \times (CaO2 - CvO2)$; calculate VO2 (O2 consumption). Normal is 3.5mL/kg/min

Ficks Diffusion: Gas thru membrane directly prop to pressure, area, & inversely to thickness/molecular wt

Hagan Pouisielle = laminar flow (velocity) thru tube; $V = [\pi r^4 \Delta P] / 8L\mu$; impt numbers are the 4 & 8.

Hagan Pouisielle also = Resistance = $(8L\mu)/ (\pi r^4)$; μ = viscosity

Henderson Hasselbalch Eq: pKa + log [Base/Acid] = $6.1 + log [HCO3/(0.03 \times PaCO2)]$

Kf is a constant, Jv is net fluid movement, ∂ is the reflection coefficient.

$MAP = SVR \times CO$; Cardiac index = CO divided by BSA; $EF = SV/EDV$, $BMI = kg/m2$

Normal Aa gradient is 5-20mmHg. It incr's with age, V/Q mismatch, pulm shunt (V/Q=0), & low SvO2.

Normal SVR = 800-1600 dynes. Normal CO = 4.5-5 L/min. Normal CI = 2.6-4.2 L/min/m2

O2 content (mL/dL) = Sat x (Hb x 1.39) + 0.003(PaO2): only tiny Δs with PaO2.

O2 delivery: $DO2 = CO \times CaO2$. Delivery decr'd by decr'd CO (hemodynamics) or CaO2 (anemia/hypoxemia)

One French = 1/3 mm. 1.3cmH20 = 1mmHg.

$P1/V1 = P2/V2$: use to find liters of gas left in E-cylinders.

PaCO2 determination = k (Vco2/V(alv). Co2 dissociation curve linear unlike oxyHb dissociation curve.

PVR equation: $PVR = (PAP - PAOP) \times 80/CO$. Normal PVR is 50-150 dynes.sec.cm-5

Starling Equation is the Oncotic/Interstitial pressure = $Jv = Kf ([Pc - Pi] - \partial [\pi c - \pi i])$.

$SvO2 = MvO2$ = Pulm art O2 = $SaO2 - [VO2 / (Q \times Hb \times 13)]$. Normal SvO2 from pulm art is 40mmHg and 70% sat.

SVR equation: $SVR=(MAP-CVP)/CO \times 80$, Normal SVR is 800 -1150 dynes.sec.cm-5

Think of V=IR (Ohm's) so then R=V/I, so SVR (resistance) = pressure(voltage)/flow(current).

$TI = LD50/ED50$; Vd = dose/plasma[…]; MAC = ED50 of Volatiles.

Total Body deficit mEq of HCO3 = ECF vol (ie 0.2xkg) multiplied by deviation of HCO3 from 24

Transpulmonary shunt estimated by dividing Aa gradient by 20mmHg yielding percentage of shunt.

Stats

1. If data are categorical, use chi square; If data are numbers/nominal -> t-test (for 2) or ANOVA for >2 variables.

2. One needs about 20 – 30 observations of each variable to compare logistic regression data.

ANOVA: Compares nominal data for >2 variables. Contrast to t-test, see above.

Asymptotic - the data never reaches zero or always approaches (but never reaches) a specified value.

Bonferroni test: used to adjust for multiple comparisons for overall error rate of 0.05. Causes power loss.

Categorical Variables: discrete data that is Nominal (cannot be ordered ie dead or alive, yes or no) or Ordinal (can be ordered, ie with >2 possible values). Use chi-square test.

Chi square test: used to calculate P-value for nominal independent & nominal dependent variables. Assumes that all outcomes are equally likely to occur.

Confidence interval (CI) – interval estimate of a population parameter. Used to indicate the reliability of an estimate. Increasing the desired confidence level will widen the CI. The higher the confidence level, the wider CI will be.

Continuous Variables: data with unlimited number of equally spaced potential values. Examples are time, dosage, age, weight, blood pressure. Use rank sum tests (non parametric substitute for t-test) comparing medians, etc.

Non parametric tests: analyze data (ordinal) not distributed normally, also can be used for continuous data.

Null Hypothesis: There is no difference between the variables in question.

Odds Ratio: ratio of odds of having risk factor if condition present vs odds of having risk factor if condition not present. If value=1 then condition is likely in both groups. If >1 then first group more likely to have event occur.

Parametric Tests: have more statistical power when the data has a normal distribution; but can be misleading if not.

Power: one minus type 2 (β) error. Strength of population size. Probability of rejecting the null, if not true.

Reference ranges are usually 2 standard deviations from the mean (ie 95% people will fall within range). P=0.05

Relative Risk: ratio of the risk of developing an outcome over developing the outcome without the risk present.

T-test: normally used to compare data sets with one or two variables that assumes normal distribution.

Type 1 Error (α) : null hypothesis is incorrectly rejected – alpha error allowance of 0.05.

Type 2 Error (β): null hypothesis is incorrectly accepted – beta error (0.20 allowance – power)

Wilcoxon Rank Sum: univariable analysis of ordinal dependent variable. T-test for abnormally distributed data.

Computers

1. Computerized records more likely to record accurate vitals (BP) than are manually recorded vitals.

3. Cardiovascular & Pulmonary Physiology & Allergy

1 CO = SV x HR; SVR=(MAP-CVP)/CO x 80; Cardiac index = CO/BSA; EF = SV/EDV.

2. Resistance is inversely proportional to the 4th power of radius. Most SVR is due to arterioles.

3. Preload = EDV. CVP is good estimate if normal heart/lungs. Otherwise need TEE or swan.

4. Cardiac output measured by swan, thermodilution, or echocardiography.

5. Frank-Starling (vol/pressure) is larger preload results in incr'd CO/SV. EF normally remains same.

6. Pulsus pardoxus (big pulse change in tidal breathing) in presence of normal CVP is tamponade or PTX.

7. Afterload determined by SVR. Majority of hypotension is due to decr'd preload or contractility…NOT SVR.

8. Baroreceptors (carotids/arch) & Chemoreceptors (carotids/brainstem/CNS) send info via CN 9 & 10.

9. Atrial stretch (Bainbridge reflex) increases HR. Dominant with blood volume is ↑ d. Baroreflex when ↓ d.

10. Cushing reflex is brady in response to incr'd ICP. Oculocardiac is V3 to CN10.

11. Coronary reserve is ability to incr flow. Heart can't incr O2 extraction. CR exhausted @90% prox stenosis.

12. PAP > 40/20 is pathologic. PCWP should be 2-12. CVP 2-8 in spontaneously breathing pt.

13. Incr'd CO decr's PVR via pulmonary distension and recruitment of more pulmonary capillaries.

14. HPV is pulm vasc response to low PaO2 (impt). It decr's shunt. PVR incr's w/hypercarbia, hypoxia, & emboli.

15. West zone 1 only develops with PP (vent but not perfused). 2&3 increasingly higher vascular pressure. 2 is Best.

16. Pulm edema if PCWP is >20. Oncotic/Interstitial pressure equation = $Jv = Kf ([Pc - Pi] - \partial [\pi c - \pi i])$

17. Normal P50 for adults is 27mmHg. Baby 22. O2 content (mL/dL) = Sat x (Hb x 1.39) + 0.003(PaCO2)

18. Most impt WRT apnea O2 is lung storage (FRC) then Hb storage. After preO2 usually 5-10 min until desat.

19. Alveolar gas equation relates FiO2 to PAO2. Normal PA02 on 100% is 500-670mmHg.

20. Normal Aa gradient is 5-10mmHg. It incr's with age, V/Q mismatch, pulm shunt (V/Q=0), & low SvO2.

21. PaCO2 = k (Vco2/V(alv). Co2 dissociation curve is linear unlike oxyhemoglobin dissociation curve.

22. EtCO2 5-10mmHg lower than PaCO2 bc anatomic dead space always present (decr'd physiologic dead space)

23. PE will cause sharp decr in EtCO2 bc vent w/o perfusion. MH causes sharp incr bc of incr'd production.

24. Central chemoreceptors (brainstem) respond slowly (15-20min) to CO2 and pH bc of BBB.

25. Peripheral chemoreceptors (carotid bodies) respond quickly to low PaO2, high PaCO2, and acidosis.

26. Central response to hypoxia is *decr'd* Vm. Luckily, response is slower than carotid body response to *incr* Vm.

27. Dopamine can inhibit peripheral chemoreceptors (caution in awake pts) and droperidol can stimulate them.

28. Droperidol issue is blocks dopamine, dystonia, EPS, arrhythmias, etc.

29. Ondine's Curse (abnormal hypoxic/hypercapnic drive) is seen in NSGY pts, premies <60wks, OSA, & obesity.

30. O2 consumption is VO2 = CO (CaO2-CvO2). O2 delivery = DO2 = CO x CaO2.

31. Total body O2 consumption: normal adult 3-4mL/kg/min, child 5-7, newborn 7-9mL/kg/min.

32. Under anesthesia in pts with anemia, increase in HR is masked and body must incr O2 extraction.

33. Need co-oximetry to tell if COHb is present and gives percentage.

34. COHb has negative inotropic effect on heart. Asthma increase's DLCO2. (counter-intuitive).

35. Cilia are on columnar cells. Type 1 alveolar cells are for gas exchange. Type 2 produce surfactant.

36. MAP = SVR x CO; Determinants of MAP therefore are preload, afterload, HR, & inotropy.

37. Autoregulated arterial systems are cerebral, renal, coronary, hepatic arterial, intestinal, & muscle circulation.

38. Pulmonary surfactant is decreased by CPB, PE, and prolonged 100% FiO2.

39. If SVT give adenosine (can cause bronchospasm) rapid IV push 6-12mg

40. FRC = expiratory reserve volume + residual volume; Study Jensen lung vol diagram.

41. Remember closing vol (capacity) is vol of lung required to keep small airways open. ↑ s w/age, obesity, smoking, etc.

42. Fetal Hb & bilirubin have NO effect on pulse oximeters. MetHb shifts oxygen dissociation curve to left.

43. With chronic A/B abnormalities, oxyHb curve resets due to altered metabolism of 2,3 DPG.

44. Acute inc of $PaCO_s$ 10mmHg will decr pH 0.08 units; HCO_3 decr's 5 mEq/L each 10mm decr of $PaCO_2$ <40.

45. For every 0.08 change in pH there is an inverse change in K of 0.5mEq/L.

46. Some intubation criteria RR> 30, PaO_2 <60, sat <75, $PACO_2$ > 50, worsening symp's, burns, CPAP failure.

47. Some extubation criteria Vc > 15mL/kg, RR<30, PaO_2 > 60 FiO_2 50%, A-a <350, pH >7.3, PCO_2 < 50.

48. PVR inversely proportional to CO via recruitment/distension of pulm vessels. PVR incr's with vasopressin.

49. PVR equation: PVR = (PAP – PAOP) x80/CO. Normal PVR is 50-150 dynes.sec.cm-5

50. Don't cardiovert multifocal atrial tachycardia (common in COPD).

51. FRC, residual volume, and closing volume all increase with aging.

52. Transpulmonary shunt estimated by dividing Aa gradient by 20mmHg yielding percentage of shunt.

53. Anatomic dead space is 2mL/kg (~150mL). Doesn't participate in O_2 exchange, so slower RR is better.

54. For every 0.08 change in pH there is an inverse change in K of 0.5mEq/L.

55. COHb t1/2 is 1 hour in patients breathing 100% FiO_2. Must order co-oximetry to test.

56. PVR inversely proportional to CO via recruitment/distension of pulm vessels. PVR incr's with vasopressin.

57. "Time constant" is "capacity/flow." For VAs, the equivalent is brain/blood partition coefficient

58. Tissue O_2 consumption decreases 8% per each degree Celsius below 37.

59. Myocardial O_2 consumption is much less with volume work (preload), then pressure work (afterload).

60. Cardiac output incr's by 100mL/min for each kg over 70kg via stroke volume (not resting HR).

61. Static compliance (lungs) = Vt / (plateau pressure – PEEP); Dynamic compliance = Vt / (peak pressure – PEEP)

62. PEEP indicated when PaO_2 <60mmHg on FiO_2 >60%. PEEP ↓ s intrapulmonary shunting but ↓ s CO.

63. Physiologic dead space = anatomic dead space + alveolar dead space

64. Physiologic dead space represents fraction of Vt that doesn't participate in gas exchange.

65. Resting coronary blood flow is 80mL/100g/min. 6% of cardiac output.

66. Cardiac O_2 consumption is 10mL/100g/min (10% of O_2 consumption).

67. Cerebral blood flow is 50mL/100g/min (20% of CO?) & O_2 consumption of 3.5mL/100g/min.

68. Adult p50 is 26.5; Neonate is 20, HbSS is 34.

69. Afterload is a systolic event (LV wall tension. SVR is a diastolic event with arteriorlar constriction & aortic runoff.

70. Non-smokers HbCO is 1-3%. Smokers 10%. If >25% then supplemental O_2 indicated.

Allergy

1. Tx anaphylaxis w/IVF, epinephrine (Gold Standard), & benadryl. Latex allergy associated with allergy to bananas.

2. Benzos and ketamine VERY unlikely to cause allergic reaction. NMBDs & abx account for >60%.

3. Antihistamines are competitive inhibitors of histamine. They do NOT inhibit release of histamine like Epi (Gold Std).

4. NMBD induced anaphylaxis due to prior exposure, cosmetics, or soaps (quarternary ammonium groups).

5. Curare causes release of histamine and sympathetic ganglion blockade.

6. Serum tryptase is marker of mast cell degranulation. Used in determination of true allergic reaction.

7. Allergen Ab complex binds to mast cells & basophils release histamine & eosinophillic chemotactic factors.

8. Other things released: leukotrienes, prostaglandin D2 (bronchoconstriction), tryptase, chymase, kinins.

9. Abx & NMBDs compete for top 2 causes of OR anaphylactic rxns. Then latex.

10. Anaphylaxis is Ag:Ab complexes bind to mast cells & basophils. Requires previous exposure to exact or similar Ag.

11. Anapylactoid rxns (not Ab mediated); the Ag binds directly to mast cells & basophils. (vanc, morphine, mannitol, etc).

12. Allergic reactions very rare for LAs (<1%). Mostly truly are only adverse reactions. Order serum tryptase.

13. Ascertain "true" allergic rxns vs unusual, unexpected, or unpleasant reactions to medications.

14. True allery: skin manifestations, facial/oral swelling, SOB, choking/wheezing, or vascular collapse.

15. Hx of shellfish or seafood allergy has NOT been linked to allergy to IV iodine contrast. But theoretically avoid.

16. Radiocontrast anaphylactoid reactions need O2, aggressive IVF, and epinephrine.

17. Major prophylaxis is steroid & antihistamine nite before & AM of surgery. 40 pred/20 pepcid/50 benadryl.

4. General Pharmacology

1. Pharmacokinetics is what body does to drug. Dynamics is what drug does to body (effect).

2. When pH & pKa of drug are the same then drug is 50% ionized. Most drugs are amines (narcotics, LAs). RNH3+

3. Acidic drugs: NMBDs. Basic drugs: local anes (weak bases), opioids, STP, methohexital

4. Albumin binds acidic drugs and AAG binds basic drugs. Carboxylic acids are uncharged when protonated (STP).

5. Large first pass effect orally: lidocaine, propranolol, digitalis, midazolam, meperidine, verapamil

6. Lung uptake lidocaine, propranolol, propofol, fentanyl, and can serve as reservoir for future release.

7. *Ion trapping* occurs in fetus w/local anes and opioids bc of low fetal blood pH = ionized form can' leave.

8. About 75% of CO is delivered to 10% of body mass (vessel rich group).

9. Majority metabolism is in liver; also in kidney, lung, GI, bile, blood.

10. Excretion primarily kidneys. Also lungs, bile, skin, GI, breast milk, saliva, and sweat.

11. Enzymatic induction (p450) by phenobarbital, carbamazepine, phenytoin, grapefruit. Inhibition by cimetidine.

12. Phase 1 rxns oxidation (p450), reduction (halogenated compds), & hydrolysis. Phase 2 is conjugation.

13. Weak acids are ionized in alkaline urine (excreted). Weak bases are ionized in acidic urine.

14. Enterohepatic circulation is impt with excretion of vecuronium and erythromycin.

15. In pharmacokinetics - Alpha phase is distribution phase. Beta phase is elimination.

16. Clearance (in mL/min) is additive & is the summation of clearance rates for liver, kidneys, etc.

17. Vd = dose of drug divided by plasma concentration. Small Vd (ND-NMBDs). Large Vd (STP/diazepam)

18. Five beta t1/2s needed for complete elimination. In Anes we are concerned w/Context sensitive t1/2s.

19. *Effect site equilibration* is time interval b/t drug concentration needed in plasma to actual drug effect.

20. GABA chloride channels are ligand gated and result in hyperpolarization.

21. G-protein coupled receptors include all adrenergic, cholinergic, opioid, dopamine, & histamine receptors.

22. Inverse agonists (aka superantagonists) produce response below baseline response measured in absence of drug.

23. Up and Down regulation is reason for adverse effects of abrupt discontinuation of meds (and tachyphylaxis).

24. If slope of *dose response curve* is steep as in MAC1=ED50 & MAC1.3=ED95; confers small therapeutic index.

25. *Therapeutic index* is LD50 over ED50. The higher the TI the safer the drug.

26. *Ceiling effect* is when incr'ing dose does *NOT* further incr therapeutic effect (ie, sideFX predominate).

27. *Time synergism* eg is when epinephrine prolongs duration of local anesthetics.

28. *Tolerance* is larger dose required to produce the same effect. Tachyphylaxis is acute tolerance.

29. *Dependence* is characterized by behavioral response to take drug for psychic effect or discomfort of its absence.

30. *Addiction* is continued seeking/use despite repeated negative consequences.

31. Racemic Mixture examples: Bupiv, Dobutamine, STP, ketamine, VAs. Non-effective isomers can cause sideFX.

32. Levobupiv is L-isomer of bupiv which is more effect w/less CV toxicity. D-ketamine has the desirable effects.

33. Benzos and opioids are synergistic. ACh displaces ND NMBDs from their alpha subunits of nicotinic receptors.

34. Grahams Law: diffusion coefficient inversely proportional to square root of molecular weight of substance.

Receptors

1. Adrenergic (NE) receptors are on sympathetic targets (fight or flight). Catacholamines are epi, NE, & Dopamine.

2. Dopaminergic (D1&D2) receptors located on BVs (dilation) and presynaptic membranes (inhibit NE release).

3. PNS cell bodies in brain stem. Post gang secretes ACh (cholinergic-R) divided into nicotinic & muscarinic.

4. Nicotinic (ACh) receptors located at most parasympathetic targets (everywhere) & in ALL autonomic ganglia.

5. Nic: @ NMJ depolarization (skeletal musc contrxn); @ Autonomic ganglion stimulates SNS and/or PNS.

6. Muscarinic (ACh) receptors located on parasympathetic targets (smooth & cardiac muscle, gut).

7. Musc: Decr HR, inotropy, constrict bronchioles, stimulate intestinal motility, relaxes sphincters (GI & bladder).

8. Alpha 1: constricts BVs, relax gut, causes salivation, gluconeogenesis, glycogenolysis, & renal Na retention.

9. Alpha 2: *inhibits lypolysis, NE & insulin release*; constricts BVs (minor peripheral), causes platelet aggregation.

10. Beta 1: cardiac chronotropic and inotropic, lypolysis, renin release.

11. Beta 2: relaxes SM (pulm, coronaries, uterus), gluconeogenesis, glycogenolysis, insulin & lactate release.

12. D1: dilates BVs (renal, coronary, and mesenteric).

13. D2: inhibits further NE release in CNS via presynaptic membrane location.

14. H1 receptors bronchoconstrict. H2 receptors (pepcid blocks) bronchodilate.

15. H2 receptors stimulate gastric acid secretion by parietal cells and have CV effects.

16. NMDA rec blocked by Ketamine, Methadone, N2O, meperidine, Namenda & tramadol; slightly by Mg.

17. Blocking dopamine receptors (droperidol) can cause acute dytonia (torticollis). Tx with benadryl.

18. Opioid rec (G-coupled) activation (CNS) causes incr'd K conductance (hyperpolarization).

19. Stimulation of opioid rec inhibits adenyl cyclase increasing cAMP, presynaptically inhibiting NT release.

20. Opioid receptors classified mu1&2, kappa, & delta. New nomenclature?

21. Mu 2 causes hypoventilation, constipation, & dependence. Delta similar. Kappa causes dysphoria.

22. Mu 1 rec cause prolactin release (women on heroin), Mu 2 rec cause resp depression, kappa = dysphoria.

5. Pharmacology Non-opioid IV Anesthetics & Other Meds

1. *PROP* has lecithin (eggs); & metabosulfite (additive) can induce sulfite allergy or reactive airways.

2. Wake up time is 8-10min, Lungs metabolize 30%, works on GABA, decr's ICP, can cause twitching.

3. Profound brady/asystole has been described in healthy adults with prop. Does NOT potentiate NMBs.

4. Reduces Vt >>RR and decr's wheezing, nausea, & upper airway response to DL (can be used alone).

5. STP & methohexital pH > 10, will precipitate with acidic drugs (NMBDs).

6. Barbs cause severe pain subQ/arterial injection with vasoconstriction (gangrene). No pain on IV inj.

7. Barbs incr porphyrins (don't give AIP). Can also induce own metabolism (p450) except Phenobarbital.

8. Methohexital cleared fast by liver (reason for revovery). STP (t1/2 = 12h) same recovery bc of redistribution.

9. Barbs could be considered anti-analgesic. Decr CBF, ICP, CMRO2, & can cause flatline EEG.

10. Barbs can protect from focal (not global) ischemia. They are direct myocardial depressants.

11. Metho activates epileptic foci, lowers seizure threshold (ECT), unlike other barbs (EEG suppression).

12. Barbs not good choice for LMA or DL w/o NMBs (propofol better). Don't reliably block tracheal response.

13. Barbs cause post induction garlic/onion taste. Rectal metho 20-30mg/kg for MR or Peds induction.

14. Propofol, etomidate, STP, & methohexital all decrease SBP, CBF, ICP, & CMRO2.

15. Diazepam has active metabolites. Midazolam doesn't & has the shortest benzo context sensitive t1/2.

16. Benzos (like most) highly protein bound (albumin).Don't affect ICP. May decr BP (in hypovolemia).

Albuterol: β2 agonist, bronchodilates, tachy (ischemia!), drives K into cells (hypokalemia), hyperglycemia.

Aminocaproic acid (Amicar) is competitive inhibitor of plasminogen activation; protects clots.

ASA: irreversible COX inhibitor, also prevents formation of thromboxane (platelet aggregation).

ASA: onset 2hrs; Analgesic, antipyretic, anti-inflammatory. Disables platelets for life (7-10 days)

Benadryl: 12.5-50mg IV, anticholinergic. drymouth, confusion, urinary retention.

Bretylium causes release of NE then inhibits further release. HTN then hypotension. Tx for CRPS1 & resistant Vtach.

Buprenophine (mixed ag/antag) resists reversal by naloxone. including respiratory depression.

Chloropropamide (interferes w/opiates) & Tolbutamide are 1st gen sulfonylureas (long t1/2). We use 2nd gen.

Cimetadine: (H2 blocker) can cause confusion, hallucinations, bradyarrythmias, hypotension, cardiac arrest.

Cimetadine: causes brady (cardiac H2 rec), delayed awakening (crosses BBB), & impairs metab (p450).

Clonidine can prevent narcotic induced muscular rigidity (suggests symp mechanism for rigidity).

Clonidine: a2 agonist, decr SNS outflow, sedative/analgesic. Intrathecal no N/V or resp depress. Rebound HTN.

Cyclosporine associated w/seizures, nephrotox, HTN...NOT pulmonary toxicity (bleomycin).

Dantrolene: 2.5mg/kg bolus, approx 1mg/kg q6 hrs for at least 24hrs. Max dose 10-30mg/kg.

Dexamethasone: 4mg IV, 0.25mg/kg, unknown mech for antiemetic effect, anal/vulvar pruritis, hyperglycemia

Dexmedetomidine is CNS alpha 2 agonist, rapid hepatic metab, minimal resp depression (awake FOB!).

Dexmet causes *No change* in most parameters: Ventilation, CBF, CMRO2, ICP, & no nausea.

Dexmet hypnosis from locus ceruleus & analgesia at spinal cord. Cons are bradycarida, decr'd BP & SVR.

Doxapram stimulates CNS, SNS, carotid chemo rec mimicking low PaO2 stimulating respiration. *Many sideFX!*

Droperidol: (sed/antiemetic, dopa & α blocker) incr's HR & decr's MAP. Tx EPS (torticollis) w/benadryl.

Droperidol: 1mg IV, dopamine (D2) antag, antiemetic, dystonia, ↓ seizure threshold, QTc prolongation.

Edrophonium does NOT decr psuedocholinesterase activity. Pavulon, Ach esterase inh, and MAOIs do.

Erythromycin inhibits metabolism (specific p450) of midazolam.

Etomidate (like metho) can induce seizure foci although ↓ s ICP/CBF/CMRO2. Myoclonus in >50% pts.

Etomidate (pH 6.9) metab via *ester hydrolysis*, 77% bound, each 0.1mg/kg provides 100sec of unconciousness.

Etomitate benefit is CV stability. Cons are adrenal cortical suppression (4-8hrs), PONV, and injection pain.

Flumazenil (10-15mg/kg IV) useful for 20 minutes (then re-sedation possible).

Guanethedine (peripheral antihypertensive) replaces nerve terminal NE. Intermittent doses - HTN (NE release).

Haloperidol: 1mg IV, dopamine (D2) antag, anitemetic/psychotic, same efx as droperidol

Hemabate: synthetic PGF2α. For uterine atony unresponsive to oxytocin & abortions. N/V/D are side-FX.

Heparin: potentiates antithrombin 3, t1/2 90min, can give FFP if pt has low Anti3 levels (impaired response).

Ibuprofen: NSAID, antipyretic. Disables platelets transiently. 5-10mg/kg in peds.

Ipratropium/Atrovent: blocks bronchial musc cholinergic rec (duonebs), doesn't cross BBB (anti-cholinergic synd)

Ket incr's ICP & SNS activity, but it's approved to tx status epilepticus. cataleptic state. Somatic pain > visceral.

Ketamine also been shown to prevent opioid induced hyperalgesia in chronic opiate therapy.

Ketamine has been shown to prevent hyperalgesia in perioperative period.

Ketamine has low protein binding (key), highly lipid soluble, min'l resp depression. Gets no GABA.

Ketamine's direct myocardial & resp depressant masked by SNS stimulation (ICU/sepsis reveals this).

Metformin is biguanide (lactic acidosis) & should hold 48 hrs prior to surgery, newer data 24hrs.

Metformin: ↑ s insulin sensitivity, assoc'd w/lactic acidoisis in pts w/CHF, renal failure, shock, etc.

Metoclopramide: 10mg IV, dopamine antagonist, GI upset, dystonia, incr LES tone, (avoid in Parkinson's).

Minoxidil (antihypertensive & hair growth) is associated with pericardial effusion, tamponade, and pulm HTN.

NSAIDS/ASA can shunt arachadonic acid to leukotrienes leading to bronchospasm in asthma pts.

Pepcid/Famotidine: (H2 blocker - 12hrs) 10mg IV in holding area, or PO night prior & AM of surgery.

Pepcid/Famotidine: H2 blocker with < sideFX than cimetidine or ranitidine.

Pitocin: synthetic oxytocin, induces uterine contraction, but other smooth muscle relaxation (↓ BP).

Pralidoxime is an acetylcholinesterase reactivator. Given w/atropine to tx organophos poisoning.

Promethazine: 6.25-25mg IV, antihistamine, sedation, decreased seizure threshold

Ranitidine: H2 blocker, bradycardia, hypotension, decr dose in renal failure.

Ritodrine & Terbutaline are beta agonists used as tocolytics in obstetrics. Nifedipine has replaced now.

Scopolamine decreases cognitive fxn in Alzheimer's. Appears like early Alzheimer's in healthy people.

Scopolamine: 1.5mg transderm, anticholinergic, drymouth, confusion, urinary retention.

Toradol IV/IM like 6-12mg morphine. Inhibits plts, renally cleared. Diclofenac IV 1mg/kg also used.

Tranexamic acid:10x more potent than Aminocaproic acid. Useful in trauma & dysfxnal uterine bleeding.

Tylenol: PO, PR at this time. Antipyretic. 10-15mg/kg in peds.

Ziconitide (25AA-peptide, selective N-type CCB) is a potent intrathecal analgesic for refractory chronic pain.

Zofran (Parkinson safe): 4mg IV, 0.1mg/kg peds, 5HT3 rec antag, dizziness, HA, QTc prolongation (also dolesetron).

1. Glucagon incr's cAMP, HR, inotropy, CO, and stimulates release of catecholamines. Tx for BB overdose (1g IV)

2. NMDA rec blocked by Ketamine, Methadone, N2O, meperidine, Namenda & tramadol; slightly by Mg.

3. Blocking dopamine receptors (droperidol) can cause acute dytonia (torticollis). Tx with benadryl.

4. H1 receptors bronchoconstrict. H2 receptors (pepcid blocks) bronchodilate.

5. H2 receptors stimulate gastric acid secretion by parietal cells and have CV effects (↑ HR).

6. BB do NOT produce orthostatic hypotension. Midazolam converts to lipid soluble once in blood.

7. GnRH superantagonist, Abarelix can medically castrate.

8. Use NSAIDs for bone pain. Morphine for cancer pain. MAOIs & meperidine can increase temp (fever).

9. MAOIs include: selegeline, phenylzine, & tranylcypromine.

10. Cause histamine release: Curare, Atra & Mivacurium, Sux. Morphine, codeine, meperidine, protamine/vanc (if rapid)

11. Metabolism: Non-specific Esterases: Remifentanil, etomidate. 2/3 atracurium

12. Metabolism: Psuedocholinesterase: Sux, mivacurium, all ester LAs.

13. Metabolism: Hoffman: Cisatracurium. 1/3 atracurium

6. Pharmacology Autonomics

1. Orthostasis (ANS dysfxn) equals decr in SBP >30mmHg & absence of HR incr when standing from sitting.

2. Central ANS is hypothalamus, medulla, & pons. Peripheral ANS is thoracolumbar (SNS) & craniosacral (PNS).

3. Autonomic ganglia contain cell bodies of postganglionic fibers (non-myelinated). Pregang (CNS) are myelinated.

4. SNS pregang fibers come from IML cell column in T1-L3 spinal cord. Symp chain is 22 paired ganglia.

5. Adrenergic (NE) receptors are on sympathetic targets (fight or flight). Catacholamines are epi, NE, & Dopamine.

6. Dopaminergic (D1&D2) receptors located on BVs (dilation) and presynaptic membranes (inhibit NE release).

7. PNS cell bodies in brain stem. Post gang secretes ACh (cholinergic-R) divided into nicotinic & muscarinic.

8. Nicotinic (ACh) receptors located at most parasympathetic targets (everywhere) & in ALL autonomic ganglia.

9. Muscarinic (ACh) receptors located on parasympathetic targets (smooth & cardiac muscle, gut).

10. Alpha 1: constricts BVs, relax gut, causes salivation, gluconeogenesis, glycogenolysis, & renal Na retention.

11. Alpha 2: *inhibits lypolysis, NE & insulin release*; constricts BVs (minor peripheral), causes platelet aggregation.

12. Beta 1: cardiac chronotropic and inotropic, lypolysis, renin release, salivation, lypolyisis.

13. Beta 2: relaxes SM (pulm, coronaries, uterus), gluconeogenesis, glycogenolysis, insulin & lactate release.

14. D1: dilates BVs (renal, coronary, & mesenteric). cAMP mediated. Only agonist we use is Fenoldopam.

15. D2: inhibits further NE release in CNS via presynaptic membrane location.

16. Musc: Decr HR, inotropy, constrict bronchioles, stimulate intestinal motility, relaxes sphincters (GI & bladder).

17. Nic: @ NMJ depolarization (skeletal musc contrxn); @ Autonomic ganglion stimulates SNS and/or PNS.

18. Termination of effect of endogenous catacholamines is reuptake, but exogenous is via diffusion.

19. Endogenous cat (NE, Epi, Dop) located at nerve terminals and adrenal medulla.

20. Synthetic catacholamines are isoproterenol, dobutamine, fenoldopam, dopexamine.

21. Epi low dose causes vasodilation/incr CO (also PVCs), hyperglyemia, greatly decr's RBF, tx of allergic rxns.

22. NE mainly a1 and b1, incr'ing SVR & improving coronary flow. Minimal b2 agonist.

23. Dopamine D1 at low doses improving blood flow. Higher doses mainly b1 incr'ing HR, releases NE stores.

24. Dobutamine incr's CO with little change in HR or SVR (decr). Good for diastolic dysfxn.

25. Isoproterenol (b1&2) incr's CO, myocardial O2 req, & decr's MAP. Chemical pacemaker. Tx's bronchospasm.

26. Fenoldopam is mainly D1 agonist incr'ing RBF & decr'ing SVR. Used mainly for HTN or vascular surgery.

27. Ephedrine indirect (both) sympathomimetic (NE). Tachyphylaxis. Watch for depletion of stores (cocaine/meth).

28. Phenylephrine direct a1 agonist (venous>arteries). Incr SVR, decr CO, HR. Longer acting than NE.

29. ACE-I: cardiac remodeling, no rebound HTN. SideFX: cough, prolonged hypoTN, hypercalcemia, neutropenia.

30. Clonidine: a2 agonist, decr SNS outflow, sedative/analgesic. Intrathecal no N/V or resp depress. Rebound HTN.

31. Prazosin is a1 antag (venous & arteries) used in CHF & pheo. Causes fluid retention & orthostatic hypoTN.

32. Minoxidil *dilates arteries only*, stims renin secretion, reflex tachy. Usually give with BB and diuretic.

33. Hydralazine *dilates arteries only*, reflex tachy, fluid retention. SideFX: SLE syndrome & hemolytic anemia.

34. CCBs potentiate NMBDs , decr HR & conduction velocity. Avoid in WPW. Nicardipine is peripheral CCB.

35. Labetalol β t1/2 is 5.5 hrs via kidneys. Oral $\alpha1/\beta1\&2$ ratio is 1:3 & IV is 1:7. Much more β block effect.

36. Contraindications labetalol: HR<60, SBP<100, CHF, bronchospasm, heart block, unstable hemodynamic pts.

37. BBs do NOT produce orthostasis or alter MAC. Nonselective BBs can cause hyperglycemia (b2 blockade).

38. Don't mix with CCBs. If OD then *give atropine first*. If persists then give CaCl & glucagon.

39. SNP *dilates arteries & veins*. Causes cyanide toxicity (tx w/thiosulfate) & MetHb (sat 85%, get co-oximetry).

40. NTG *dilates mainly veins*. Metab in BVs to NO-> cGMP -> vasodilation. Causes MetHb and incr'd ICP.

41. Inhaled NO relaxes pulm vasculature with minimal systemic effects. Metab'd to nitrate in blood by Hb.

42. Adenosine dilates coronaries and decr's inotropy. Give 6mg IV for paroxysmal supraventricular tachy.

43. Anticholinergics: Atropine/scopolamine (tertiary amines, mydriasis) & glyco (quarternary, antisialagogue).

44. Give physostigmine (crosses BBB) for tx central anticholinergic syn (emergence delirium) in PACU.

45. Edrophonium short acting anticholinesterase used in dx of M. Gravis.

46. Endogenous catacholamines have no oral bioavailability bc are conjugated & oxidized by GI & Liver.

47. Dopamine interferes with carotid bodies and resp drive. Can inhibit release of insulin-> hyperglycemia.

48. Extravasation of catacholamines causes intense vasoconstriction. Tx with phentolamine (α1&2 blocker)

49. Pts on antihypertensives have incr'd response to direct sympathomimetics & decr'd response to indirect.

50. During 1st 20 days of TCAs or MAOIs ephedrine will have exaggerated response bc incr'd endogenous NE.

51. Don't give meperidine to MAOIs bc can cause HTN crisis, convulsions, and coma.

52. H1 receptors bronchoconstrict. H2 receptors (pepcid blocks) bronchodilate.

53. H2 receptors stimulate gastric acid secretion by parietal cells and have CV effects.

54. Ritodrine b2 agonist IV in pregnancy, inhibits contrxns. SideFX: Hypokalemia, hyperglycemia, tachycardia.

55. Phenoxybenzamine: blocks α1>α2. Causes hypotension. Most commonly used in treatment of pheo.

56. Phentolamine non-selective α blocker. Used in acute hypertensive emergencies (also intra-op pheo removal).

57. Meto/Atenolol: long acting β1 blockers, both proven to decr death post MI, target HR 50-70.

58. Non-selective BB: Propranolol, Nadolol, Labetalol. Prone to cause hyperglycemia & bronchoconstriction.

59. Selective BB: Metoprolol, Atenolol, Esmolol, Bisoprolol. Remember there's still small amt of b1 rec in periphery.

60. Digitalis (Afib tx): inhibit NaKATPase, prolongs AV conductance, positive inotropy.

61. Digitalis toxicity causes: hypokalemia, hypothyroid, hypomagnesemia, hypercalcemia.

1. Epinephrine – ↑ s HR, inotropy, BP. Arrythmogenicity not seen until doses are >0.12-0.18 mcg/kg/min. HR less responsive in elderly & CAD. At doses <0.12 mcg/kg/min there is ↓ SVR & ↑ EF. No inotropic improvement w/very high doses (leads to stronger a1). Gets a1, a2, b1, b2. 1-2mcg/min b2, 4mcg/min b1&2, 10-20 mcg/min alpha & betas. Also drug of choice for life threatening allergy. Starting dose 0.01 mcg/kg/min.

2. Norepi – primarily a1 but some b1&2 effects. Spesis tx with 0.01mcg/kg/min. Great for increasing SVR with compensatory ↓ in HR. No effect on chronic pulm HTN but can ↑ PVR in pts w/acute pulm HTN. Starting dose 0.01 mcg/kg/min.

3. Phenylephrine – only a1. ↑ s SVR at expense of CO/CI. Can ↑ cardiac index in sepsis via ↓ HR, also ↓ s lactic acid & ↑ s UOP. Dose range from 0.3-3mcg/kg/min. Causes ↑ in PVR so if pulm HTN, then norepi better. Starting dose 0.3 mcg/kg/min.

4. Isoproterenol – pure b1 & b2 agonist. 1-5 mcg/kg/min. Vasodilates mesenteric vascular bed. ↑ RBF & ↓ SVR & MAP. Stimulates sinus node stopping bradycardia. ↑ s HR & ↓ s afterload. ↑ s CO but ↓ s DBP & can cause RV ischemia. ↓ s pulm HTN & bronchospasm. Used as chemical pacemaker.

5. Dopamine – a1, a2, b1, b2, DA1, DA2 agonist. Mostly b1 3-10mcg/kg/min so ↑ HR. At low doses 1-3 mcg/kg/min

the DA1's vasodilate coronaries, renal, & mesenteric vessels. Not renoprotective as once thought. Used in CHF & ↓s PVR. Good for improving diastolic function. Very high doses (>10mcg/kg/min) will get α1 constriction. Dysrythmogenic bc evokes release of endogenous NE stores.

6. Dobutamine – b1 (mainly), b2, α agonist. Incr's contractility and SV. Decr's SVR, PVR, & CVP. Good for severe CHF from 2-10mcg/kg/min, higher doses make no difference. HR more less unaffected. Good for diastolic function as is dopamine. Dopamine vs dobutamine main difference is incr'd HR with Dopamine. 1-15mcg/kg/min. Mix with D5W (like dopamine) to avoid inactivation by alkaline solution.

7. Fenoldopam – D1 & D2 agonist. No adrenergic properties. Decr's SVR & Incr's RBF. Use doses of 0.01-0.8mcg/kg/min for renal protection in vascular anesthesia. Contra in glaucoma. Use for aortic cross clamp AAA.

8. Dopexamine – b2>>b1 (10x) & DA1, DA2 ag. ↑ HR & inotropy. ↓s SVR, CVP, MAP. Non-arrythmogenic.

9. Milrinone – PDE inhibitor, incr's cAMP improving Ca ion flow. ↑s contractility & ↓s SVR main actions. Also decr's PVR (tx pulm HTN). Bolus doses of 25, 50, or 75mcg/kg ↑s the cardiac index & SV. Improves LV diastolic fxn. May need alpha agonist to counteract hypotension. Primary indication is short term tx of CHF & pulm HTN.

10. Vasopressin: ADH; potent vasoconstrictor (40unit IV push) in ACLS VFib. Constrict splanchnic bed in hypovolemic shock, increasing SVR. Give 1-2 units IV bolus to assist in decr SVR.

11. Amiodarone: class 3 antidysrhythmic, prolongs action potential phase 3 of cardiac cycle. 150-300mg IV.

12. Lidocaine: for PVCs, Vtach; 1-1.5mg/kg q 3-5 min with max dose ~ 300mg.

13. Procainamide: for PVCs, Vtach; 100mg IV q5-10 min

14. Atropine: 0.5 mg IV q2 min to total dose of about 2mg. Peds 20mcg/kg each dose.

15. Adenosine: 6mg IV push then 12mg, then another 12 if needed to convert SVT.

16. Glucagon incr's cAMP, HR, inotropy, CO, and stimulates release of catecholamines. Tx for BB overdose. Mechanism is independent of adrenergic receptors aside from it inducing catecholamines.

17. SNP *dilates arteries & veins*. Causes cyanide toxicity (tx w/thiosulfate) & MetHb (sat 85%, get co-oximetry).

18. NTG *dilates mainly veins*. Metab in BVs to NO-> cGMP -> vasodilation. Causes MetHb and incr'd ICP.

7. Pharmacology Volatile Anesthetics

1. Fluorination provides more stability, less toxicity, and more resistance to metabolism (des/sevo/iso).

2. Halothane sensitizes the heart to arrhythmogenicity of catecholamines and causes hepatic necrosis.

3. Methoxyfluorane can cause high output renal failure due to incr'd levels of inorganic fluoride.

4. Enfluorane can cause seizure activity as well as accumulation of fluoride ions.

5. Isoflurane (1980) less metabolized & quicker on/off than predecessors (not sevo/des). Very pungent odor.

6. Sevo/Des halogenated exclusively with fluoride. Very fast on/off.

7. Immobility measured by MAC (1.0 prevents movement 50% pts). MAC 1.3 for 99% of pts. MAC bar 1.5.

8. CNS enhancing of inhibitory channels (hyperpolarization) involves GABA and Chloride ions.

9. CNS blocking of excitatory channels (prevents depolarization) involves Na channels.

10. N20 incr's skeletal musc tone, expands gas spaces, diffusion hypoxia. Sympathomimetic via catecholamines.

11. Keep sevo at 2L if procedure > 2 MAC hrs to prevent rebreathing of compound A (nephrotoxic in animals).

12. CO2 absorbent temp inrc's with degradation (especially sevo) when dessicated (also causes C monoxide prod).

13. MAC unaffected by gender. Decr'd by pregnancy and anything decreasing mentation (ie old, intox, hypothy).

14. End tidal conc approximates PA and Pbr. Incr'd PI speeds onset (concentration effect) only possible w/N20.

15. Second gas effect independent of conc effect. Mostly effective with N20 and O2. Alveolar hyperoxygenation.

16. Rate of incr of PA is higher with hyperventilation and decr'd venous return (or decr'd CO).

17. Speed induction (gas): low B/G coefficient, R to L shunt, Decr'd CO/venous return, incr'd Vm, PI, & fresh flow.

18. V/Q mismatch does NOT influence rate of induction with volatile agent.

19. Brain/blood time constant for iso 4 minutes. Sevo/des 2 min. Equilibration =3 time constants (6-12 minutes).

20. N20 has very low BG coefficient (0.46) so will enter gas filled spaces (middle ear, GI, cranium, bullae, etc).

21. Metabolism only impt for halothane/methoxyfluorane (more soluble). NOT impt for iso/des/sevo.

22. Des/sevo/iso <5 min 50% decrement time. After 6 MAC hrs 90% decrement 14min/65min/86min respectively.

23. Des/sevo/iso incr HR. Des >1 MAC stim SNS & mildly incr's EF. Cardiac index/CO not affected (unlike halo).

24. Volatiles prolong QT and sevo should be avoided in pts with LQTS. Mainstay tx of LQTS is b-blockers.

25. Anes preconditioning of heart is direct protection & enhancement of ischemic precond'ing (via Katp channels).

26. Volatiles decr FRC, Vt, response to hypoxic/hypercapnic resp drive, and increase RR.

27. Volatiles only minimally inhibit hypoxic pulmonary vasoconstriction.

28. Des/iso cause airway irritation (cough, spasm, breath holding) ONLY at 1 MAC or greater.

29. N2O incr's CMRO2 and CBF. Halo/des/sevo/iso decr CMRO2 & if > 1MAC then incr CBF, ICP, and decr CPP.

30. Volatiles do NOT abolish cerebrovascular responsiveness to changes in PaCO2.

31. Volatiles increase latency and decrease amplitude of SSEPs and decr reliability of MEPs.

32. Sevo and Enflurane show eplileptiform activity on EEG.

33. Halo/iso/des produce trifluroacetate via hepatic metab can lead to immune rxn hepatic necrosis. Liver dz okay.

34. Use Iso in neuro bc increase CSF absorption but doesn't stimulate secretion. p109 hall

35. Use Sevo in neuro bc increases CBF less than Des and Iso.

36. Amount of VA taken up in 1st minute is equal to amt b/t squares of any numbers (min) thereafter. P30 hall

37. Isoflurane at <1 MAC causes NO change in CO due to compensatory incr HR. It incr's RAP & decr inotropy.

38. Iso can produce coronary steal (vasodilation of normal coronaries). Emergence is 8min per MAC hour.

39. Increase in rate of rise (FA/FI) ratio speeds inhalation induction except in R to L cardiac shunt.

40. Keep Sevo @ 2L/min (some sources 1L/min) reduces rebreathing of compound A (formed from absorbant).

41. Dessicated baralyme favors formation of compound A. Dessicated soda lime opposite.

42. Iso and Des incr HR at < 1MAC. Sevo decr's HR until 1MAC and then increases it.

43. Des decreases cardiac index at 1MAC. Iso has no change at 1MAC.

44. Vessel rich group receives 75% of CO. Brain receives 20%. Kidneys receive 20%. Coronaries receive 6%.

45. Fluoride induced nephrotoxicity (DI) manifests by inability to conc urine (via inhibtion of adenylate cyclase).

46. Main stem intubation causes incr rate of rise of FA/Fi & decr'd rate of rise in arterial partial pressure of gas.

47. Sudden doubling of cardiac output increases volatile uptake by 2x. But slows induction? (WTF dershwitz).

48. Barometric pressure (ie Denver) is inversely proportional to VA uptake. So higher up = slower uptake.

49. MAC increased by hypernatremia. MAC unaffected by thyroid dz, duration of anesthesia, or gender.

50. Amount of VA taken up in 1st minute is equal to amount b/t squares of any numbers thereafter. P30 hal

51. Lipid solubility (oil/gas partition) correlates w/MAC. 150 divided by MAC approximates the coefficient.

52. A mixture of 2 volatile anesthetics would be termed an azeotrope (mixture that can't be easily separated).

53. Severe anemia would ↓ blood:gas partiion speeding inhalation induction and causing faster awakeing.

54. VAs do NOT provide analgesia. Def'n of pain includes "experience" so controversial when "deep."

8. Pharmacology Opiates

1. Opioid rec (G-coupled) activation (CNS) causes incr'd K conductance (hyperpolarization).

2. Stimulation of rec inhibits adenyl cyclase increasing cAMP, presnaptically inhibiting NT release.

3. Receptors classified mu1&2, kappa, & delta. Newer nomenclature?

4. Mu 2 causes hypoventilation, constipation, & dependence. Delta similar. Kappa causes dysphoria.

5. Rec's found in CNS & periphery, but beneficial effects are in sub gelatinosa (Rex lam 2) of spinal cord & CNS.

6. Neuraxial opioids do NOT cause sympatholysis, weakness, or loss of proprioception. Visceral specific.

7. Neuraxial opiois can cause n/v, pruritis, urinary retention, resp depression, and activation of latent viruses.

8. Systemic absorption of epidural (not spinal) opiate is similar to equal dose given IM.

9. Coughing or straining (but not body position) can affect spread of opiate within CSF.

10. Women show greater potency and slower onset with opiates than males (gender specificity).

11. Breathing is slow and deep. Cerebral vasocontrictors so decr's CBF and possibly ICP. Can decr MAC by 50%.

12. Opioids do NOT alter NMBDs response. Somewhat synergistic effect (sedation/resp depression) with benzos.

13. Potency: Morphine 1: Alfenta 25: Fentanyl 100: Remi 250: Sufenta 1000. Meperidine is 0.1 (less potent).

14. M6G is active metabolite that accumulates in renal failure. Morphine causes histamine release.

15. Fentanyl rapid infusion can cause stiff chest syndrome (tx w/NMBs). Also bradycardia, but CV very stable.

16. Biliary spasm pain (post op) differentiated from angina w/naloxone (doesn't relieve angina). NTG relieves both.

17. N/V caused by direct stimulation of *dopamine receptors*. IM causes more N/V. Medulla is N/V inhibitory.

18. Opioid tolerance requires 25 days whereas dependence may occur after 2 days.

19. Long-term opiate use (miosis & constipation persist) can produce immunosuppression, as can abrupt withdrawl.

20. Meperidine gets kappa rec (shivering). Can cause seizures (normep), orthostasis, & serotonergic syn.

21. Alfenta 1/3 duration of axn/onset (90sec) of fentanyl. Similar to remi (80sec). Very lipid soluble. Ok in ESRD.

22. Remi context sensitive t1/2 is 4 minutes. Metabolized by non-specific plasma esterases (like etomidate).

23. Morphine IV onset 10-20 min, peak 30, duration 4-6 hrs. Causes histamine release.

24. Buprenorphine, butorphenol, nalbuphine, & pentazocine are agonist/antagonists. Less sideFX & dependence.

25. Tramadol synthetic opiate w/efficacy like Tylenol#3. Blocks reuptake of NE & serotonin < resp depression.

26. Naloxone (shortest of the 3) given 1mcg/kg IV increments reverses resp depression (works or 30-45min).

27. Nalmefene (longer t1/2) is used like naloxone. Can be given IV, IM, or even subcutaneously.

28. Natrexone is used orally for *maintenance tx of opioid addicts* and for ethanol abuse (blocks pleasant effects).

29. Methadone (t1/2 15-30h) is longest acting opioid with less withdrawl symptoms and is used in cancer pain.

30. Morphine PO 30mg = 10 IV/IM = 0.1 Epidural = 0.01 intrathecal.

31. Morphine 10mg IV = Dilaudid IV 1.5mg = Demerol IV 75mg = Methadone IV 10mg

32. Morphine 30mg PO = Dilaudid 7.5mg = Demerol 300mg = Oxycodone PO 30mg = Hydrocodone PO 45mg

33. Mu 1 rec cause prolactin release (women on heroin), Mu 2 rec cause resp depression, kappa = dysphoria.

34. Codeine (2-3%) is metabolized to morphine. 300x less affinity for mu receptor than morphine

35. Hydrocodone (Lortab, Norco) is metabolized to hydromorphone (dilaudid).

36. Ziconitide (25AA-peptide, selective N-type CCB) is a potent intrathecal analgesic for refractory chronic pain.

37. Morphine is NOT metabolized in CP450 but by glucuronidation.

9. Pharmacology NMBD

1. Need for relaxation is for DL, surgical optimization, & facilitating mech vent. Not analgesic/amnestic.

2. Nicotinic Ach-r is ligand gated. Decr's membrane potential -90 to -45mV. ACh metabolism is 15msec.

3. Neostigmine is ACh-esterase blocker AND stimulates presynaptic replenishment of ACh stores.

4. ACh-r's have 5 units with ACh binding the 2 a-subunits. EJRs replace gamma with epsilon unit.

5. EJR proliferation resists ND NMBDs and causes excessive incr in K with sux.

6. Sux (0.3ED95) onset 30-60 sec dur 5-10min. Phase 2 block (TOF <0.3) with bigger doses.

7. Sux metab by psuedocholinesterase 75% b4 reaching NMJ. Increases K by 0.5-1mEq/L.

8. MG is auto attack ACh-r, decr'ing #. Hypersensitive to NDs and resistant to sux. Eaton more sensitive to BOTH.

9. Dibucaine inhibits pseudo by 80%. Homo-atypical 20%. Hetero 55%. Reflects quality not quantity of pseudo.

10. Burns, crush, or denervation injury don't give sux 24 hrs p injury. EJRs peak p 7 days; decr 6 mos post injury.

11. FDA limits sux in children bc of subclinical MD (usually recognized by age 6).

12. Atropine IV (not IM) and priming (w/ND) decr's sux induced cardiac dysrrhythmias (not incr K).

13. Pts with renal failure have normal hyperkalemic response to sux, can be safely given. Caution sux in ICU pts.

14. Sux does NOT incr ICP (does incr IOP). Gastric pressure can be offset by priming dose of ND NMBD.

15. ND NMBDs are large, highly ionized, & H20 soluble. NOT orally available & do NOT cross BBB or placenta.

16. Renal Dz alters pancuronium & vec. Others can be eliminated by liver, bile, pseudo, and/or Hoffman.

17. Enhance ND NMBDs: VAs, aminoglyocides, LAs, antiarrythmics, dantrolene, Mg (OB!), Li, tamoxifen, & MG.

18. Resist ND NMBDs: Calcium, corticosteroids, phenytoin. Also burn & CVA pts bc of EJRs.

19. Histamine w/ atra, miva, & sux(mild) -> hypoTN/tachy. NOT pancuronium (atropine-like at cardiac musc-R).

20. NMBDs should be used max of 2 days to prevent myopathy lasting weeks to months.

21. NMBD induced anaphylaxis due to prior exposure, cosmetics, or soaps (quarternary ammonium groups).

22. Pan (0.07ED95) onset 3-5 min dur 60-90 min. Increase HR via vagolytic effect (see above).

23. Vec (0.05ED95) onset 3-5 min dur 20-35 min. Hepatic, biliary, renal excretion.

24. Roc (0.3ED95) onset 1-2 min dur 20-35 min. RSI dose duration = pancuronium. Largely biliary excretion.

25. Atr (0.2ED95) onset 3-5 min dur 20-35 min. Laudanosine (metabolite) stimulate CNS. 1/3 hoffman 2/3 ester

26. Cis (0.05ED95) onset 3-5 min dur 20-35 min. Tiny laudanosine. 1 of 10 stereoisomers of atra. 100% hoffman.

27. Miv (0.08ED95) onset 2-3 min duration 12-20 min. Short bc 2/3's metabolized by psuedocholinesterase.

28. Obicularis oculi response better approximates laryngeal response using ND NMBDs. *Ulnar with sux.*

29. TOF ratio is 4th twitch over 1st twitch. 0.7 normal/unrecognizable. 0.3 is phase 2 block w/sux.

30. Reverse if sustained tetanus (5 sec), head/leg lift (5 sec), or tongue depressor test.

31. Even if TOF no fade = 70% rec can be blocked. Even if Vt is 5ml/kg 80% receptors can be blocked.

32. Neostigmine max dose 0.07mg/kg, allow 15-30 min for full antagonism. Hypothermia lengthens blockade.

33. Sugammadex encapsulates steroidal NMBD, reversing (roc/vec), & have no CV effects. Not FDA approved.

34. NMBDs don't stop heart bc bind nicotinics (not musc). SA & AV nodes have adrenergic and muscarinics.

35. Dibucaine of 80 is normal, 40-60 Heterozygous, & 20 is homozygous for atypical psuedocholinesterase.

36. Pralidoxime is an acetylcholinesterase reactivator. Given with atropine to tx organophos poisoning.

Phase 1 Block (depolarizing): no fade, TOF ratio = 1, no post-tet potentiation, no reversal.

Phase 2 Block (non-depolarizing): fade, potentiation, TOF > 0.7 adequate for reversal.

Phase 1 block enhanced by AcHesterase drugs and shows NO post-tetanic potentiation.

Obicularis Oculi degreee of paralysis approximates diaphram. Psuedocholinesterase t1/2 is 12hrs.

Hypokalemia (flaccid paralysis) decr's NDNMD dose requirement, but incr's reversal needed.

Hypo/hyperlemia doesn't affect MAC.

Cause histamine release: Atra, Miva, & Sux. Morphine, protamine. NOT Doxacurium.

All anticholinesterase drugs also inhibit psuedo. Sux prolonged after NDNMBD reversal.

Vecuronium will cause paralysis in NMS, but not in MH. Oral dantrolene causes muscle weakness.

Sux induced tachy is due to nicotinic adrenergic ganglionic stimulation.

NMS (dopamine depletion) tx'd by bromocryptine, amantidine, and Dantrolene. NO predilection to MH.

CP (20% decr'd MAC): sensitive to sux, resistant to NDs. Not susceptible to hyperkalemia despite EJRs. 2009B ACE.

10. Pharmacology Local Anesthetics

LAs block transmission of action potential via voltage-gated Na ion channels. Block Na ion conductance.

LAs prevent achievement of neural threshold potential and do NOT alter resting transmembrane potential.

Most predictable effective block via good concentration of LA at 3 successive node of Ranvier.

Ropivicaine and Levobupivicaine are single enantiomers (not racemic mixures).

Repeated depolarization produces more effective binding of LAs: *Use dependent* or *frequency dependent* block.

The lower the pKa , the greater the percent of un-ionized fraction (works best) at a given pH.

Grahams Law: diffusion coefficient inversely proportional to square root of molecular weight.

Most LAs are weak bases (base = non-ionized, conjugate acid = ionized).

Benzocaine pKa is 3.5 so exists as a neutral base under physiologic conditions.

Other LAs pKa 7.6-8.9 so < ½ unionized in body. Stored as salts that are acidic (for stability).

Acidic salt storage (vials) of LAs is reason bicarb added sometimes to increase the unionized fraction.

LAs work poorly in acidic environments (ie abscesses or infection). Too much ionization (don't work).

Lipid solubility varies directly with potency and duration of action. Inversely w/latency (time of onset).

Max dose infiltrated lidocaine 300mg. Bupivicaine 150mg. Ropivicaine 200mg.

Max Local: Lido w/o epi 5mg/kg; Lido w/epi 7mg/kg. Bupiv 2.5mg/kg. Ropiv 2mg/kg.

Greatest plasma concentration post block: intercostal > caudal (gavity) > epidural > brachial plexus > fem/sciatic.

Etidocaine gives much more motor blockage than bupivicaine.

Type A alpha: myelinated; large motor, proprioception, fast conduction

Type A beta: myelinated; small motor, touch, pressure, fast conduction

Type A gamma: myelinated; muscle tone, fast conduction

Type A delta: myelinated; pain, temperature, touch, fast conduction

Type B: myelinated; preganglionic autonomic

Type C: unmyelinated; dull pain, temperature, touch, slow (unmyelinated) conduction

LAs are vasodilators, the most vasodilatory being tetracaine (hence most prolonged by epi during spinal).

Ester LAs undergo hydrolysis. Amides metab by liver. Lungs help w/lidocaine, bupivicaine, and prilocaine.

Epi usually added as 1:200k (ie 5mcg/mL). Lengthens duration; does not help with onset.

CNS toxicity (circumoral numbness, tinnitus, seizures, coma) most common. Usually due to vascular injection.

CV toxicity (arrhythmias, collapse) less common. HypoTN, QT prolong, QRS widening. Bupivicaine bad.

Allergic reactions very rare for LAs (<1%). Mostly truly are only adverse reactions. Order serum tryptase.

Procaine earliest injectable LA. Spinal causes higher incidence of nausea.

Tetracaine common in spinal anesthesia. High risk of TNS. Rarely for epidural or PNBs.

Tetracaine metab is slow even though its ester. 1/10th as fast as chloroprocaine. High motor blockage differential.

Chloroprocaine (use bisulfite free) used for short axn epidural. Fastest metabolized, interferes w/opioids

Lidocaine (only achiral LA) most versatile. Cauda equina syn (CSA) & TNS (SAB).

Mepivicaine similar to lidocaine. Less vasodilation and slightly longer duration of action.

Prilocaine has rapid metab and low acute CNS toxicity (40% < lidocaine). But metabolite induces metHb.

Bupivicaine "fast in, slow out", near zero TNS. Cardotoxic. Do not use 0.75% for epidural bc IV inj possible.

Ropivicaine is a single enantiomer similar to bupivicaine but less potent & much less cardiotoxicity.

Levobupivicaine is single S (-) enantiomer of bupivicaine. Very similar to Ropiv but much less popular.

Eutectic mixture (EMLA) uses lidocaine and prilocaine for topical use. Takes 30-60min to work.

Increased TNS w/lithotomy position, knee arthroscopy, & outpt status. NOT conc, epi, or needle size.

Cauda equina syndrome is persistent neurologic deficits usually caused by CSA with lidocaine.

TNS sx's within 12-24 hrs. Most resolve within 3 days. Some persist >1wk. NSAIDs first line tx.

TNS is dysesthesia or severe pain. NOT associated with sensory/motor loss, bowel, or bladder dysfxn.

Meperidine has local anesthetic properties. Structure similar to atropine ($\uparrow$ HR), & metabolite causes seizures.

Intralipid 20% given 100mL IV (1.5mL/kg bolus) removes LAs from their binding sites on cardiac muscle.

Intralipid initial bolus followed by infusion 0.25mL/kg/min for 10-60 min. Bolus can be repeated 1-2x if asystole.

11. Pathophysiology and Anesthesia: Neurologic, Neuromuscular, & NM Blockade

1. Normal CBF is 50mL/100g/min (15% of cardiac output). Brain 1.4kg (700mL/min) & has no O2/glu stores.

2. CBF and CMRO2 (coupled) directly proportional. VAs cerebrodilate (incr CBF) but decr CMRO2 (uncouple).

3. SEVO incr's CBF the least. ISO is decr's CMRO2 the best. VA's incr in ICP is offset by hypocapnia.

4. CBF decr's 1mL/100g/min for every 1mmHg PCO2 under 40 (for 8 hrs). Doesn't last bc CSF HCO3 incr's.

5. CPP = MAP-ICP (or CVP) the greater. 50 mmHg is normal. CBF autoreg bt MAP 50-150 (even with pressors).

6. Autoregulation has 1-3 minute lag time so spikes are bad.

7. Above 1 MAC, VAs abolish autoregulation (bad). IV anesthetics do NOT.

8. If PaO2 drops below 50mmHg, then CBF increases exponentially.

9. Benzos decr CMRO2 and CBF like other IV anesthetics. Opioids decr CBF (maybe ICP) & ?CMRO2.

10. Clonidine and Dex have no effect on ICP but can decr CPP via decreasing SVR.

11. Normal ICP is 10-15mmHg. If >15 avoid ventilatory depressants bc can incr PCO2 an thus ICP.

12. No evidence of benefit if PaCO2 <30. Avoid PEEP b/c can incr ICP (impairs cerebral drainage).

13. Mannitol (1g/kg) lasts 2-4 hrs. If given rapidly can incr ICP. Lasix works but less effective.

14. If sitting position need CVL and precordial Doppler (VAE >25%). TEE most sensitive for dx.

15. VAE symptoms are like PE with cyanosis and mill wheel murmur (late sign).

18. Cord transections at risk for hypoTN/hypotherm. Within symp chain autonomic dysreflexia (persist HTN).

19. Autonomic dysreflexia (8% of cord injuries above T6): HTN, bradycardia, cutaneous vasodilation.

20. Cerebral vasospasm common 3-15 days after SAH. Tx with HHH and Nimodipine (CCB).

21. HHH: hypertesion, hemodilution, hydration to normovolemia (used to be hypervolemia).

9. ECT seizures need to be at least >20 sec for therapeutic. Propofol shortens and etomidate lengthens.

10. Generally no ECT with intracranial mass lesions. ICDs not affected by ECT.

11. Hypercapnia can increase the seizure threshold. Parasymp (tonic) then Symp (clonic).

Normal CBF is 50mL/100g/min. Will incr by 1mL/100g/min q1mm Hg incr in PaCO2.

If incr ICP can use trimethophan to control BP on DL & intubation. Induces mydriasis, rarely used.

Brain O2 consumption is 3.5mL/100g/min of brain tissure vs cardiac is 10mL/100g/min of cardiac tissue.

Nitrous oxide decr's amp w/NO effect on latency. Etomidate incr's BOTH. Barbs and VAs dec amp & incr latency.

MEPS affected by VAs and IV anesthetics. Fentanyl doesn't affect as all.

Spinal shock (initial 6wks) is precursor to autonomic hyperreflexia (HTN due to stimulus below injury level).

Reverse steal is when nl vessels constrict (w/Decr PaCO2) shunting blood to ischemic areas.

At > 2 MAC cerebral autoregulation is abolished. We usually keep VAs MAC between 0.5 & 1.0 in neuro cases.

Gabapentin excreted unchanged by kidneys; not metabolized.

Posterior ION more common perioperative than anterior ION. Associated w/prolonged prone spine surgery.

Spinal shock (1-3wks) :bradycardia, hypotension, no temperature regulation below level of lesion.

Maintain CPP above 70. All IV anesthetics are potent cerebral vasoconstrictors, but ketamine cerebrodilates.

Intraocular pressure incr'd by acidosis, hypercarbia, acute HTN, hypoxia, valsalva.

All anticholinesterase drugs also inhibit psuedo. That's why sux longer after NDNMBD reversal.

Normal CBF 50ml/100g/min. EEG changes at 22, isoelectric at 15, & irreversible neuronal death at 6.

Persistent intraoperative hyperventilation (decr CNS HCO3) leads to spont resp at lower PaCO2.

Cholinergic crisis is differentiated from MG crisis by edrophonium "worsening" the cholinergic crisis.

Sux induced tachy is due to nicotinic adrenergic ganglionic stimulation. Brady due to direct musc on heart.

Levodopa (Parkinson's) can lead to hypoTN, arrythmias. βt1/2 is 6-12hrs, can have rebound rigidity, cont' periop.

MEPs very sensitive to VAs. Use TIVA, keep Hb at 10, avoid hypotension to ensure good cord perfusion.

ICP ↑ d: TIVA, < 0.75 MAC of VAs, hyperventilation (temporary), steroids (long term), analgesia, MAP >70.

Neuromuscular Disease & Blockade

Phase 1 Block (depolarizing): no fade, TOF ratio = 1, no post-tet potentiation, no reversal.

Phase 2 Block (non-depolarizing): fade, potentiation, TOF > 0.7 adequate for reversal.

Phase 1 block enhanced by AcHesterase drugs and shows NO post-tetanic potentiation.

ACh action at NMJ terminated by hydrolysis by acetylcholinesterase rather then by diffusion!

Potentiate NMB: VAs, LAs, anticholinesterases, abx (not erythro, PCN, or cephlasporins), dantrolene, CCBs, Mg.

Potentiate NMB (more): hypocalemia, hypokalemia, hypothermia, acidosis/alkalosis, lasix, ketamine, Li.

Resist NMB: Burns, hypercalcemia, hyperkalemia, paralyzed extremity.

Large doses of Neostigmine (>5mg) can independently cause NM blockade.

Extubate after stable vitals, circulation, strong grip, 5 ec head lift, tongue out, etc. See ext criteria in Critical care.

Botox (neurotoxin) prevents release of ACh at nerve terminal (dependent on calcium influx).

Don't give sux 10-60days post massive burn. May need increased amounts of ND NMBDs.

Dibucaine inhibits pseudo by 80%. Normal is 80. Homo-atypical 20. Hetero 55. Reflects quality not quantity.

Nerve stimulator *negative* electrode should be more distal for maximal response. Negative = Distal.

Muscular dystrophy (x-linked) incr's risk of MH. Muscles are hypertrophied bc of fatty infiltration.

Duchene's die (15-25yo) because of CHF or pneumonia. Assess cardiac status. Usually discovered by age 6.

Myotonic dystrophy causes impaired relaxation of muscle (atrophy, weakness).

Myotonic dystrophy (auto dominant) – spinal does NOT ensure relaxation (Bier block does). Avoid sux!

FDA limits sux use in children bc of subclinical or unrecognized NM dz, not bc of MH risk.

Myasthenia autoimmune to ACh receptors. Proximal weakness. 25% associated with thymoma.

Eaton-Lambert autoimmune to Ca-influx channels at NMJ preventing ACh release. Small cell lung cancer.

Myasethenic Syndrome (Eaton Lambert) more sensitive to BOTH NMBDs.

Huntington's chorea patients have decr'd levels of psuedocholinesterase.

In MS pts avoid sux (incr's K) & SAB. LEA is acceptable. MS exacerbated by SAB!!! NOT LEA or PNBs.

NMS (dopamine depletion) tx'd by bromocryptine, amantidine, and Dantrolene. NO predilection to MH.

Vecuronium will cause paralysis in NMS, but not in MH. Oral dantrolene causes muscle weakness.

Atropine does not affect nicotinic synapses (NMJ – motor unit).

12. Pathophysiology and Anesthesia: Cardiovasular (also see Autonomics Pharm) & ACLS

1. Most periop MIs occur 48-72 hours post op.

2. HR >110 most likely to lead to ischemia. If >105 for 5 min's incr risk of death 10 fold.

3. Cont BB, CCB, nitrates, ACE, & statins or incr'd mortality. Hold hypoglycemics & diuretics.

4. ST depression >1mm = ischemia. Most sensitive for ischemia is TEE wall motion abnormalities.

5. Periop MI risk reduced to 5-6% @ 6 mos out. Risk stratification NOT superior to H&P & risk reduction therapy

6. If pt has >2 risk factors for CAD give periop long-acting BB or clonidine day of surgery.

7. Cardiac index > 2.5L/min/m2 and/or EF of >55% is considered good cardiac function. CI is CO/BSA.

8. Minimize hemodynamic changes to DL with <15 sec duration, topical or IV lido 1.5mg/kg.

9. Only long-acting BB (meto) have been shown to decr cardiac risk, NOT esmolol.

10. Phenyl improves coronary PP AND *benefit* offsets any incr in myocardial O2 requirements.

11. MS – keep HR low/nl, SVR incr'd and avoid head down and other causes of pulm HTN.

12. MR – causes magnitude relative V waves on PA cath. Keep incr HR, decr SVR. Pancuronium good.

13. AS – angina w/o CAD due to LVH. Keep HR 60-100, know tardus/parvus,. defib ready. CPR ineffective.

14. AR – angina w/o CAD due to LVH. Wide pulse pressure, keep incr HR and slight low SVR.

15. MVP – avoid incr SNS activity, sitting postion, incr'd cardiac emptying. Can lead to eventual or acute MR.

16. If >6 PVCs/min, 3+ sequential, or on T wave give IV lido and correct underlying cause.

17. V-tach is wide QRS and >120 bpm. If good perfusion give lido, amio, or procainamide. If not, DC cardiovert.

18. WPW is pre-excitation along Kent fibers with short PR, wide QRS, & delta wave. Avoid SNS and CCB.

19. Prolonged QT syndrome treated with BB or left stellate gang block. Avoid droperidol.

20. Give IHSS (septal hypertrophy) phenylephrine. Don't give B-agonists or potent vasodilators (NTP).

21. Nitrous oxide can cause pulm HTN and decreases inspired O2 concentrations.

22. For severe cor pulmonale/RVF can give b-agonist & milrinone for synergism vent improvement/vasodilation.

23. If cardiac tamponade, induce with ketamine with spont vent. Definitive tx is pericardial drainage or death.

24. Metabolic requirements are decreased by 8% for every degree below 37 Celsius.

25. At 30 degrees the normal contracting heart uses 8-10mL O2/100g/min.

26. Cardioplegia induced hyperkalemia can cause heart block and decreased myocardial contractility.

27. Most common cause for difficulty weaning from CPB is decr SVR. Watch K, Ca, Mg, Glu, pH, & dysrhythmias.

28. Protamine causes histamine release ->hypo and pulm HTN. IDDM may have incr risk for protamine rxns.

29. Desmopressin improves platelet fxn in patients with Von Willebrands Dz.

30. If B-agonists needed during Off-pump CABG distal anastamosis, then CPB should be considered.

31. Resting coronary blood flow is 80mL/100g/min. 6% of cardiac output.

32. Cardiac O2 consumption is 10mL/100g/min (10% of O2 consumption).

33. Cerebral blood flow is 50mL/100g/min (20% of CO?) & O2 consumption of 3.5mL/100g/min.

34. Curare causes release of histamine and sympathetic ganglion blockade.

35. IABP is foundation for management of acute cardiogenic shock (massive MI/pump failure).

1. EKG hyperkalemia: PR markedly prolonged, QRS broadened, ST elevated, and T-waves peaked.

2. EKG hypokalemia: PR & QT prolonged, ST depressed, T wave flat, & maybe *U-wave* present.

3. EKG hypercalcemia: prolonged PR, widened QRS, short QT interval.

4. EKG hypocalcemia: prolonged QT interval

5. EKG hypomagnesemia: prolonged QT interval

6. EKG WPW: (pre-excitation along Kent fibers) short PR, wide QRS, & *delta wave*. Avoid SNS & CCB.

6. Nitroprusside can cause coronary steal (art & vein) and cyanide toxicity (tx'd by Na thiosulfate).

7. Use lidocaine for ventricular arrhythmias. Metabolized by liver.

8. Procainamide 1 gram loading dose (100g/5min) for supraventricular and ventricular arrhythmias.

9. Procainamide (1.5mg/kg) suppresses ventricular ectopy when lido is ineffective.

10. NaHCO3 indicated when: pre-existing hyperK, trycylic OD, to alkalinize urine, or late in CPR.

11. Esmolol for Afib with RVR, metabolized by RBC esterases.

12. Amiodarone lengthens action potential, slowing rate thru nodal tissue, 150mg loading.

13. Amiodarone increases the refractory period & reduces membrane excitability in the heart.

14. Essential hemodynamic parameters are HR, Preload, SVR, PVR, Inotropy, & myocardial compliance.

15. The lower the dicrotic notch on a-line tracing, the lower the SVR and visa versa. SVR=[(MAP-CVP) x 80]/CO

16. Normal SVR = 800-1600 dynes. Normal CO = 4.5-5 L/min. Normal CI = 2.6-4.2 L/min/m2. Normal PVR 50-150.

First degree AV block: PR >0.2 sec; can be caused by quinidine, digitalis, BBs, MI, congenital, etc

Second degree AV block type 1: Wenckebach; progressive PR length until dropped QRS.

Second degree AV block type 2: sudden dropping of QRS without prelude.

Third degree AV block: atrial beats unrelated to ventricular beats. Complete block; vent rate 20-40.

LBBB implies cardiac disease (CAD, HTN, LVH). RBBB does not & is usually not significant.

Pulseless arrest (absence of BP despite cardiac activity): 80-90% of people will have v-fib on EKG.

BLS: ABCs, jawtrust, CPR; 1 cycle = 30:2 for >8yo, 15:2 for <8yo. No AED on <1yo.

BLS: adult compression depth 1.5-2 inches, peds 1-1.5 inches, infants 0.5-1 inch.

PALS: initial defib is 2j/kg, then 4j/kg, none if <1yo. O2 first! Atropine 20mcg/kg, epi 10mcg/kg.

ACLS: tachy w/pulse >150, unstable (CP, CNS, shock) -> sync cardiovert (SC)

ACLS: pulse >150, stable wide QRS (>0.12s) -> amio 150mg IV, if torsades (give Mg 1-2g), or SC

ACLS: pulse >150, stable narrow QRS, regular -> 6mg adenosine push, may repeat x2, nodal agents

ACLS: pulse >150, stable narrow QRS, irregular -> nodal agents (dilt, beta blockers)

ACLS: Brady (<60 unstable), if poor perfusion -> transQ pacing, atropine 0.5-3mg, epi 2-10mcg/min

ACLS: Brady (<60 unstable), if poor perfusion -> tx cause, prepare for transvenous pacing.

ACLS: pulseless, shockable (VT, VF) biphasic 200j, mono 360j, then 5 cycles CPR (2min)

ACLS: pulseless, non-shockable (PEA, Asytole), 5 cycles CPR (2min). pulseless meds

ACLS: pulseless meds, CPR (2min), 1mg epi q3-5min, vaso 40u x1, atropine 1mg q3-5min (max 3mg)

ACLS: other meds, Amio 300mg then 150, Lidocaine 1-1.5mg/kg (max 3mg/kg), Mg (1-2g) over 10min

ACLS: other meds, NaHCO3 only late (1mEq/kg IV), Procainamide (refractory VF) 100mg IV, q5min.

ACLS: H's: Hypovolemia, hypoxia, hypoglycemia, hypo/hyperkalemia, hypothermia, H+ (acidosis).

ACLS: T's: Toxins, tamponade, tension ptx, thrombosis (PE or MI), trauma.

ALCS: d/c CPR after evidence of brain death or cardiac unresponiveness (approx 5-10min).

ALCS: meds down ETT: NAVVEL: Naloxone, atropine, vasopressin, valium, Epi, Lido

ACLS: ETT meds give 2.5x the IV dose in 10ml diluent. IV and IO obviously preferred.

13. Pathophysiology and Anesthesia: Pulmonary

1. *Asthma* causes reversible expiratory airway obstruction/inflammation and bronchial hyperresponsiveness.

2. Status asthmaticus tx'd with IV steroids (gold std), inhaled b-agoniss, & possibly general anes.

3. GETA: avoid ketamine, histamine (sux ok), DES, PEEP. Pretx with nebs, IV lido, maybe deep extubate.

4. For bronchospasm deepen VA, give albuterol, IV steroids, check for mechanical obstruction.

5. *COPD* is FEV1/FVC < 70%. Severe is FEV1 < 50% of predicted. Know BODE index.

6. Anes: ABG, ?PFTs, use small tidal vol, slow RRs. Chronic hypercapnia should not be corrected.

7. *Pulm HTN* is mean PAP > 25 at rest. Severity indices are dyspnea, hypoxia, syncope, met acidosis, RV failure.

8. Right heart cath gold std for dx of pulm HTN. Worsened by acidosis, hypercarbia, hypoxia, & vasopressors,

9. Manage by maintaining preload, minimize tachycardia, avoid hypoxemia/hypercapnia (incr PVR).

10. Intraop can give NO (10ppm), inhaled prostacyclin, or milrinone (PDE inhibitor). Parturient mortality is 50%!

11. *OSA* can cause chonic HTN (systemic and pulmonary) via chronic decr in PaO2 during apneic episodes.

12. Neck circumference more impt than BMI wrt severity of OSA. BMI alone is most impt risk factor for OSA.

13. If morbidly obese, severe OSA, or suspected Pickwickian syndrome, get pre-op ABG & mimic values intraop.

14. For *lung resection* if FEV1 or DLCO are < 40% predicted by lung perfusion scan -> advise against surgery!!

15. If exercise study <10ml/kg/min (decr O2 consump) predicts 25-50% mortality -> advise against surgery!!

16. Always suggest stop smoking at ALL times. Benefit (decr'd post-op pulm complcxns) only shown at 4-6 wks.

17. Right sided DLTs most often inserted too deep deflating RUL. Use FOB for placement.

18. Use BB (bronchial blocker) if post op ventilation required b/c don't have to switch to SLT.

19. For R sided BB insert deep so cuff herniates into RUL bronchus. Insert deep if L sided also to prevent moving.

20. Use peds FOB with ARNDT BB with 8mm ETT. Use loop with FOB and inflate BB cuff 6mL.

21. Univent has built in BB. Rotate ETT to select which bronchus desired to block.

22. Volatile anesthetics do NOT afftect regional hypoxic pulmonary vasoconstriction.

23. Ventilate depdt lung with 100% O2 at 8-10mL/kg preventing atelectasis. Keep same Vm by increasing RR.

24. OLV desat?: Check DLT, recruit maneuver, CPAP non-depdt lung, PEEP depdt, clamp pulm art, resume 2LV.

25. For mediastinoscopy watch for ptx, hemorrhage, brady (vagal stretch), and inominate artery compression.

Some intubation criteria RR> 30, PaO2 <60, sat <75, PACO2 > 50, worsening symp's, burns, CPAP failure.

Some extubation criteria Vc > 15mL/kg, RR<30, PaO2> 60 on FiO2 50%, A-a <350, pH >7.3, PCO2 < 50

Normal vital capacity is 70mL/kg, so ~5L is normal. Anatomic dead space is 2mL/kg (~150mL).

Respiratory quotient = CO2 produced divided by O2 consumed. Fat=1. Carbs=0.8, Protein=0.7, Normal diet=0.84

Bleomycin pulmonary toxicity (irreversible fibrosis) risk is increased by high FiO2 during surgery.

PFTs indicated for all tracheal resections. Carinal tumor may be absolute contraindication.

Resp alkalosis results in hypokalemia leading to decr'd capture in pacemakers (incr'd threshold).

Transplanted lungs lack normal cough reflexes (predispose to pneumonia).

Acute respiratory failure defined as PaO2<60 despite O2 support (FM) in absence of R->L intracardiac shunt.

14. Pathophysiology & Anesthesia: Endocrine/Metabolic & Liver

Endocrine/Metabolic

Insulin isolated in 1922. Causes glu uptake, storage of glycogen, stops lypolyis & ketogenesis.

IDDM - < 20 yrs old, peak incidence at puberty, loci at chromosome 6. NIDDM - < 40 yrs old, 90% are obese.

Gestational DM – glucose intolerance 2-3% of pregnancies. Resolves post partum

Secondary DM – pancreatic resection, or insulin resistance via beta blockers or phenytoin, etc.

Insulin resistance via impaired stimulation of tyrosine kinase on insulin receptors. This is reversible thru diet.

Impaired glu tolerance (insulin elevated but not measured) masks prediabetics (bc glu levels normal).

DM: Glucocorticoids and placental somatotropin (HPL) increase insulin resistance.

DM: Counter regulatory hormones (epi, glucagon, GH, NE, cortisol) are increased resulting in ketogenesis.

High dose insulin regimens (>100u/day) are atherogenic. Elderly more at risk for HONK (>350 mOsm).

HbA1c (ie sugar coated Hb) is average glu over 3 months. Goal is < 7.5%. Non-diabetics have < 6.05%.

Reg insulin: onset 30min, peak 3hr, duration 6hr. NPH: onset 2hrs, peak 6hr, duration 12hr.

Preop dose is usually 2u regular insulin SQ q 50 over 150 glu. Or can give 5u IV if >250.

Tx for DKA: IVF, IV regular insulin, K replacement (insulin drives K intracellular).

Hypoglycemia (<50) CNS, renal dysfxn. seizures, diaphoresis. Tx 25-50mL D50. Glucagon 2mg IM/IV.

DM: Pts likely have retinopathy, nephropathy, CAD (risk equivalent), orthostasis, & neuropathies.

DM: vagal denervation, ↓ temp, brady resp's only to epi bc ANS dz, A/O stiffness, gastroparesis, scleroderma.

DM: if giving a lot of LR remember lactate convert to GLU, ↑ insulin req. VA's inhibit insulin secretion.

Treat insulinoma with surgery or streptozocin as well as BB & phyentoin. All ↑ insulin resistance.

Metformin is biguanide (lactic acidosis) & should hold 48 hrs prior to surgery, newer data 24hrs.

Chloropropamide (interferes w/opiates) and Tolbutamide are 1st gen sulfonylureas (long t1/2). We use 2nd gen.

Hyperthyroidism (Graves, iatrogenic) shows weakness, tachycardia, anxiety, wt loss, ↑'d temp.

Hyperthyroidism: beta-receptors have increases sensitivity.

Hyperthyroidism: *thyroid storm* is CHF, dehydration, shock. Happens 6-18hrs post-op. Can mimic MH.

Hypothyroidism: lethargy, hypothermia, diastolic HTN, ↓'d CO & metabolic rate

Hypothyroidism: *myxedema coma* (opposite of thyroid storm) is hypothermia, hypoventilation, CV collapse.

Asymptomatic thyroid dz rarely affects anesthesia. Hyperthermia can ↑ MAC 5% per degree above 37.

Hyperparathyroid (↑ Ca) unpredictable responses to NMB. Mostly resists ND NMBDs. Sux variable.

DiGeorge (thymic hypoplasia): Hypocalcemia, micrognathia, neonatal tetany, vascular abn (TOF).

Acute hypocalcemia shows Chvostek's (face spasm) or Trosseau's (carpal spasm) sign.

Hypocalcemia (ie parathyroids inadvertently removed) sx's occur 24-72 hrs later (laryngospasm).

Hypercortisolism (Cushing's): obese, tx signs & symptoms (glucose, electrolytes, etc).

Hypocortisolism (Addison's): hypotension, hypoglycemia, hyponatremia, but HYPERkalemia.

Hypocortisolism (Addison's): wt loss, weakness, adrenal insufficiency, need stress dose steroids.

Serum cortisol returns to normal levels 1-2days after surgery. 5-25mcg/dL is normal level.

Daily cortisol secretion 30, minor surg 50, major surg 75-150, high stress 150-300.

Hyperadosteronism (Conn's): from tumor, hypokalemia, HTN. Tx with K and Spironolactone.

Pheo: HTN, headache, impending doom. Common in MEN1A, 2B, and VHL.

Pheo: give PO alpha blocker 10-14 days prior to surgery. NO beta blocker in absence of alpha blockade.

MEN2a med thyroid Ca & hyperparathyroidism. MEN2b pheo, medullary thyroid Ca, & neuromas.

VHL associated with hemangiomas of CNS and pheo. Stanozolol is one tx of hemangiomas.

Acromegaly: ↑ d airway soft tissue, long mandible, neuropathy, DM, thick skin, large tongue.

Acromegaly: Test for ulnar circulation (poor in this dz) prior to radial a-line.

Diabetes Insipidus (DI): (↓ ADH) give DDAVP (intranasal) or ADH (IM) 2 days prior to OR.

Fluoride and Lithium make kidney unresponsive to ADH (nephrogenic DI)

SIADH (↑ ADH): hyponatremia, restrict PO fluid intake, can give demeclocyline.

Central Pontine Myelinosis: rapidly correcting hyponatremia causes this fatal neurologic disorder.

Liver

Anemia (via renal failure) contributes to ↓ d oncotic pressure & volume overload (CHF & ascites).

Direct (conjugated) bilirubin elevated due to hepatocellular dysfxn or biliary tract obstruction.

Elevated in liver dz: AST/SGOT, ALT/SGPT, & LDH. If Alk phos think biliary dz.

Elevated plasmaglobulin characterizes autoimmune hepatitis.

ESLD: contraindication to elective surgery. Up to 50% mortality.

ESLD: infuse glu containing solutions preoperative. Impaired degradation of insulin, glycogen depletion.

ESLD: less protein, less clotting factors (except 8), less glucose (no storage), ↑ unconjegated bili (steatorrhea).

ESLD: use glucose containing solutions, proein supplements, TPN, B12, vit K, folic acid.

Esophageal varicies travel to azygous and hemi-azygous veins to heart.

EtOH have liver enxyme elevations in ratio of 2:1, AST/ALT. Think Alcohol (ALT) is the base.

Factor def'cy and thrombocytopenia (hypersplenism). Vit K def'cy bc lack of bile production.

Hepatic encephalopathy: obtundation, asterixis (flap), fetor hepaticus (liver breath), impaired immunity.

HypoTN in carcinoid tx'd w/somatostatin bc epi/ephedrine can cause release from tumor (worsening).

Indirect (unconjugated) bilirubin elevated due to hemolysis, CHF, Gilbert's, or Criglar Najjar.

Intrapulmonary shunting occurs secondary to portal HTN (cirrhosis).

MEDS highly cleared by liver: versed, digitalis, propranolol, meperidine, Amides LAs

Psuedocholinesterase t½ is 14 days. Only low in SEVERE liver disease. All VAs ↓ hepatic blood flow & perfusion.

Serum albumin <3 gm/dL suggests chronic (not acute) liver failure. Albumin long t1/2 = 21 days.

The only "real" LFTs are albumin & PT. All others are tests for liver destruction.

Vecuronium/pancuronium undergoes significant hepatic metabolism (not others).

Wernicke-Korsakoff: seen in alcolholism thiamine deficiency -> confusion, ataxia, nystagmus

15. Pathophysiology and Anesthesia: Hematologic

Hemostasis

1. Vascular injury exposes TF (endothelium), which binds F7. That complex activates 9, 10, etc.

2. Local thrombin separates F8 & vWF, cleaves fibrinogen to fibrin, & activates F8 to crosslink fibrin.

3. Protein C inactivates F5&8, S potenitates C. Anti-thromb, heparins, alpha macro, & TFPI limit coagulation.

4. Heparin's anticoagulant effect is from increasing activity of antithrombin & thrombomodulin.

5. Plasmin cleaves fibrin & fibrinogen, leading to D-dimers & FDPs which inhibits thrombin.

6. Surgery & massive trauma are hypercoaguable states bc of acute phase reactants.

7. Bleeding time is test of plt fxn (independent of coag factors) & poor predictor of surgical bleeding.

8. Factor 7 deficiency only would have prolonged PT but normal PTT. F7 t1/2 is shortest at 6 hrs.

9. ACT is time in seconds for whole blood to clot in test tube. Normal 90-120 sec. CPB want > 400.

10. Coagulation factors <30% of normal or plt count of < 50k can cause uncontrolled bleeding.

11. vWF made in endo&megakaryocytes & stored in plts. *vWBDz* also have decr in F8. Tx w/DDAVP & FFP.

12. Don't give DDAVP with CAD bc big vWF multimers can cause plt aggregation leading to MI.

13. Cryo has high conc of F8, vWF, F13, & fibrinogen. In *HemoA* give DDAVP first, then cryo, F8, FFP.

14. DDAVP induces release of stored vWF and F8 into plasma. Give to HemoA and vWBDz.

15. F8 (endothelial cells) & 4 (Ca) not produced in liver. Levels (8) can be low in Rheum A. & Ulcerative C.

16. Lupus anticoagulant more likely to be associated with thrombosis than hypocoagulability

17. Impair plt fxn: EtOH, ASA, NSAIDS, uremia, multiple myeloma, infused dextran & hespan.

18. DVT/PE associated w/ F5 Leiden, MTHFR (incr homocysteine), decr'd protein C&S and antithrombin.

19. DIC is syndrome with low plts, incr'd D-dimers, F8 low. Severe liver dz looks similar, but F8 levels not low.

20. If heparin resistance, give FFP to provide antithrombin for heparin to act on.

21. Fondaparinux is a single pentasacharride of LMWH given QD. Decr'd risk of HIT & incr'd risk of bleeding.

22. Direct thrombin inhibitors (argatroban) are used in HIT. Or you can use plasmapheresis to clear antibodies.

23. Argatroban metab by liver (avoid in liver dz). Lepirudin cleared by kidneys (avoid in renal dz).

24. Surgery or puncture of non-compressible vessels contraindicated 10 days after TPA.

25. There is a temporary hypercoaguable state after *initiation* of warfarin bc of quickly decr'd protein C.

26. There is a temporary hypercoaguable state after *d/c* of warfarin bc of decr concentrations of TPA inhibitor type1.

27. Know ASRA guidelines. Most frequent Q is wait 24hrs after "BID/wt based lovenox" is given b4 neuraxial.

28. Cryo if isolated fibrinogen <125mg/dL. Reverses Urokinase. Not as prevalent due to newer factor concentrates.

29. Prolonged PTT associated w/Hemo A, B, & vWBD. HemoA have elevated PTT in all but the mildest disease.

30. Blood doesn't coagulate in tissue bc of endothelial prostacyclin (I2) & macrophage scavenge of clotting factors.

31. Thromboelastography (dynamic test of clotting): stong clot creates -> thick TEG, weak -> thin TEG.

32. Hemophilia A (80% of hemophiliacs) has low concentrations of factor 8. X-linked recessive (only males).

33. Hemophilia B (20% of hemophiliacs) has low concentrations of factor 9. X-linked recessive (only males).

34. Hemophilia C (rare) has low concentrations of factor 11. Auto recessive, but heterozyogotes can have sx's.

35. In hemophilia A, give DDAVP first, then F8 conc (factor concentrates), then FFP or cryo.

36. VW Dz: (↓ d vWF, ↓ d platelet adhesion): also has ↓ in F8. Tx w/DDAVP & FFP, cryo last. Plts don't help.

37. DDAVP induces release of stored vWF and F8 into plasma. Give to HemoA & vWBDz.

38. DDAVP is contraindicated in type 2B vWB patients, very low vWF levels (thrombocytopenia).

39. Aminocaproic acid (EACA) prevents formation plasmin (prevents clot breakdown). Used in CPB & bleeding dz.

40. Urokinase (declotter) can be reversed by whole blood (preferred), pRBCs, & cryoprecipitate.

IVF

1. Clinically evaluate IVF vol: HR, BP, MAP, orthostasis, ABG (base excess), BUN/Cr, Hct, CVP (6-12), UOP.

2. Ketamine directly depresses myocardium manifested by paradoxical hypotension after giving to CHF/shock pts.

3. Positive pressure ventilation (PPV), valsala, sympatholysis, GA, decrease preload.

4. Need to replace deficit, maintenance, and loss (3rd spacing, exposure, blood & urine loss)

5. Use isotonic IVF 4:2:1 calculation for deficit and maintenance. Maintain UOP at 0.5-1mL/kg/hr.

6. Use 3 (minimal), 5 (chole), & 7 (trauma/bowel resection) mL/kG/hr. Replace 3:1 isotonic for EBL.

7. 4x4 holds 10mL, lap holds 100-150mL of blood. Intravascular t1/2 of NS (crystalloid) is 20 minutes.

8. NS more hypertonic (308) & acidotic (pH 5.6) than LR (273). LR causes alkalosis bc lactate metab to HCO_3.

9. Large volume NS leads to hyperchloremic non-anion gap metabolic acidosis.

10. Don't use glu/dex solutions bc risk of hyperglycemia & cerebral acidosis. Hypoglycemia is risk of d/c'ing TPN.

11. Albumin (t1/2 16hrs) is from humans but has no risk of HIV/HepB/C trans. Some Jehovah's witness refuse.

12. Hespan (t1/2 17 days) is semisynthetic d-glucose polymer that cause pruritis & is implicated in coagulopathy.

13. Dextran 40 improves microvascular circulation (plastics graft survival). D-70 used for volume expansion.

14. If > 1L (or >20mL/kg) Dextran decr's plt aggregation. Hespan decr's F8/vWF, impairs plt fxn, & incr's PTT.

15. Dextrose 5% in water (D5W) can cause hemolysis (via osmotic gradient).

16. Parkland is 4mL/kg x BSA burned for 24h fluid replacement. First ½ in 8 hrs, then remainder in next 16 hrs.

17. TBW is 60% of kg. Of that 60%, there is intracellular (55), interstitial (40), and intravascular (5).

18. ECF = 0.2 x kg. ICF = 0.4 x kg. Plasma volume is 5% of total body water. (0.6 x kg x 0.05).

19. T½ of albumin in plasma is 20 days. NaCl 3% is to be infused no faster than 100ml/hr.

20. Abrupt d/c of TPN causes hypoglycemia/tachycardia. Watch for CVL change without checking placement.

21. Fluid losses are due to evaporative, 3rd spacing, and blood loss. Use crystalloid with end pts = BP, HR, and UOP

22. Can give albumin 5-20mL/kg. If you give too much pt can get hypernatremia.

23. Most common intra-op bleeding diathesis is dilutional thrombocytopenia.

24. End-Stage Liver IVF: use glucose containing solutions bc no storage, production, & ↓ d insulin degredation.

Blood Therapy

1. Type specific matched blood ABP-Rh chances of hemolytic rxns to only 1/1000 units.

2. Type and screen (screened for common Ab) has rxn limited to 1/10,0000 units. Renew xmatch q 72 hrs.

3. Blood storage time 3-5 wks with 70% RBC viability 24 hrs after transfusion. Plt storage is 5 days at 22C.

4. One unit (Hct 70-80) ↑ Hb by 1g/dL. pRBCs have ↓ 'd clotting factors. LR can clot b/c of Calcium.

5. Whole blood is more likely to cause citrate intoxication than pRBCs.

6. Always give blood if Hb <6 g/dL or if >30% of total blood volume lost quickly (ie 2L).

7. Give platelets if count is < 50k. One unit will incr plt count 5-10k. Usually come in 6 unit packs.

8. Bacterial contamination via blood products is most likely with platelets bc stored at 20-24° instead of 4°.

9. After giving desmopressin for HemoA (↓ 'd 8), if unresponsive or fibrinogen low, give cryoprecipitate.

10. Leading causes of transfusion related death are TRALI > ABO mismatch > infectious transmission,

11. CMV most likely transmission (via pRBCs) bc not tested for. All others <1:1 million chance.

12. Stored blood has decr'd Ca, pH, and 2,3 DPG. Has incr'd K, however not clinically relevant.

13. Citrate (added) binds Ca & causes hypocalcemia & metabolism to HCO3 leading to alkalosis.

14. Give FFP (10-15mL/kg) to restore clotting factors to 30% (adequate).

15. Transfusion rxns can mimic MH except hemoglobinuria instead of myoglobinuria and EtCO2.

16. Hemolytic rxns occur via complement system (ABO wrong). Check urine & plasma for free Hb.

17. Presence of infxn or malignant disease @ operative site *contraindication* for cell saver use.

18. With normovolemic hemodilution give blood back in opposite order removed. Not intuitive.

19. pRBCs -> give for Hb <7, Hb<8 if symptomatic, acute blood loss w/hypovolemia, & if Hct <40% in pulm dz.

20. EBV is 95, 85, 75, 70mL/kg for premie, newborn, >3mos, and >1yr respectively. Calc MABL or order labs.

21. Massive transfusion defined as 1 or + blood vol. Cplcxns: dilution, DIC, ↓ temp, pH, Ca, ↑ K, glu, volume

22. FFP has all components exccept pRBCs. Give for bleeding 2° to doc'd factor defcy or after massive transfusions.

23. Calc the dose (FFP) by estimating the plasma volume: TBVx(1-Hct) then multiply by 25% (factor level needed)

24. Rapid administration of FFP will cause transient hypocalcemia & ↓ BP. It may transmit pathogens.

25. Cryoprecipitate: has high conc of F8, vWF, F13, & fibrinogen. must have 150 mg fibrinogen & 80 IU F8.

26. Cryo Indications: in hemo A after DDAVP given, isolated low fibrinogen, last measure in vWB Dz.

27. Platelets: Indications are <50k OR <100k in presence of active bleeding. Give premature if <100 bc risk of ICH

28. Approx 5-10mL/kg should ↑ plt count 50-100k. In adults 1unit ↑ s by 5-10k. That's why we give 6-pack.

29. Platelet storage is 5 days at 22C. Reason platelets can transmit syphilis.

30. Dilutional thrombocytopenia most com'n intraop coagulopathy. pRBCs have 20-30% of factors present.

31. First to fall after massive pRBCs is fibrinogen (give FFP or cryo), then 5&8, then platelets.

32. Frozen blood (not 4 degrees, but < -64) can be stored for up to 10 yrs.

33. PRBCs stored for 35 days with CPD-A: ATP, glucose (energy), and saline. RBC life is 120 days, Plt 10days.

34. Type & Screen: Ab's. Rh system has D, C, c, E, e, etc & Rh D is most common; must renew q 72 hrs.

35. First phase of crossmatching detects ABO, MN, P, and Lewis. 2nd Phase Rh. 3rd Phase Kell, Duffy, other.

36. Rh+ blood given to Rh- mothers (isoimmunization) can/will cause future erythroblastosis fetalis.

37. Dextran (not Hetastarch) can interfere with crossmatching of blood.

38. Under anesthesia, hemolytic transfusion rxns seen via hypoTN, Hb urea, and bleeding (not fever).

39. Na bicarb given for acute hemolytic transfusion rxn to alkalinize urine prevents precipitation of hematin.

40. Compatibility is reversed for plasma products (FFP/Cryo). AB universal donor, type O is universal acceptor.

41. ABO match is not strictly necessary for plasma products, but cyro is when possible.

42. MetHb doesn't bind O2, test with co-oximetry. Occurs with SNP, NTG, Prilocaine, and silver nitrate.

43. Each gram of Hb can carry 1.34ml O2. If Hb 15g/dl, O2 content ~ 20ml/100ml. O2 reqt at rest ~ 300ml/min.

44. With no Hb PaO2 of 100mmHg (0.003 x 100mmHg), CO 5L/min O2 delivery only 15ml/min. Grossly inadequate.

45. With Hb of 15 & CO of 5L/min, O2 delivery to tissues at rest is ~1000 ml/min: a huge physiologic reserve.

46. TRALI most common cause of transfusion related death & occurs w/FFP or platelets.

47. FFP has all components (including antithrombin 3, 5, 8, etc) except pRBCs.

48. Type and Screen takes 5 minutes. Type and Crossmatch takes 45 minutes.

49. During storage whole blood depletion of clotting factors order is plts, then fibrinogen, then 5, then 8.

50. During storage pRBCs depletion is factor 1, then 5, then 8, then platelets.

16. Pathophysiology and Anesthesia: Renal/Urinary & Electrolytes

Renal/Urinary

CKD: can be relatively asymptomatic & K […] maintained WNL until GFR is <10% of normal.

CKD: prolonged effects of insulin. Aldosterone secretion ↑ s. Hypoglycemia in diabetic surgical patients.

CKD: Can ↑ K, Mg, Cl, acidosis, anemia, uremic osteodystrophy (bone demineralization – cants excrete phosphate).

CKD: Uremic syndrome includes N/V, anorexia, pruritis, anemia, fatigue, coagulopathy.

CKD: BUN is good indicator of severity of uremic syndrome. Tx with protein restriction.

CKD: Uremic bleeding (coags normal) must order bleeding time (↓ s plt aggreg). Tx with DDAVP, cryo, epoetin

CKD: Uremic motor/sensory neuropathy can mimic restless legs syndrome, but has weakness.

CKD: Uremic pericarditis common in severe CRF. Atrial dysrhythmias common (due to metabolites/electrolytes).

CKD: Preop K should not exeed 5.5. K release is not increased however. Treat coagulopathy with DDAVP.

CKD: Defasiculating dose does not ↓ K release. Normal is 0.5 – 1.0.

CKD: Decreased proein binding results in ↑ d unbound (active) drug.

CKD: Prudent but no evidence to avoid sevoflurane (compound A & fluoride nephrotoxicity).

CKD: Annual mortality risk on HD is 25% due to infections and sepsis.

CKD: Metabolite of atra and cisatra is laudanosine (causes seizures). Its cleared by kidneys – oops.

CKD: Neostigmine is excreted 50% by kidneys so protective of reversal. ↓ dose by 50% in ESRD.

ARF: if FeNa <1 or BUN:Cr ratio >20 then prerenal cause. Give IVF challenge (1L) then lasix 100mg.

ARF: If urine has incr'd Na (>40) but decr'd osmolality (< 260), it suggests ATN (intrinsic).

ARF: causes – dehydration, pressors, cyclosporine, toradol, immune rxn, rhabdo (large particulates).

Fenoldapam (D1 & alpha2 agonist) ↑ s UOP and lowers SBP, but no evidence that benefits ARF.

Ca Oxalate (65%) & struvite (20) make up 85% of renal stones. Others are uric acid, cystine, CaPO4.

Hepatorenal syndrome is acute oliguria with decompensated cirrhosis. Jaundice, ascites, ↓ RBF&GFR

TURP syndrome is IVF shifts &solute Δs leading to hemolysis, cerebral edema, renal, pulm edema, HTN.

Bladder perforation can cause shoulder pain from diaphragmatic irritation.

Glycine (bladder irrigation fluid) toxicity can result in transient blindness, delayed emergence, & death.

ESWL more at risk for hypotension (on emergence from bath) associated with regional anesthesia.

ESWL can cause lung injury/hemoptysis, arrythmias, and EKG artifact.

Renin/angiotensin/aldosterone system activation leads to renovascular HTN.

Decrd RBF releases renin -> Ang I -> Lungs/Ang2 -> adrenal aldosterone -> retain Na & H20

ADH incrd by VAs, fluid loss, and positive pressure ventilation. . Reason for post-op hyponatremia.

ANP causes vasodilation, decr'd Na & H20 retention, prevents release of renin and aldosterone.

BUN incrd by protein, GI bleed, dehydration, trauma, preg.

GFR decr's sharply at MAP < 50. Renal autoregulation between MAP of 60-160mmg Hg.

Rapid infusion of mannitol can cause Incrd ICP (causes vasodilation) and decrd SBP.

VAs decr RBF and GFR and therefore UOP. RBF is 20% of CO.

FeNa = (UNa/PNa) / (UCr/PCr) x 100%. FeNa <1 = Pre-renal. If >1 then tubular damage.

Fractional excretion of urea nitrogen = FeUN = (UNa/PNa) / (UCr/PCr) x 100%. Pre-renal if <35%. ATN if >50%.

Electrolytes

Tx hypercalcemia with 1L NS (dilution), bisphosphonate, disodium etidronate, calcitonin, HD.

Tx hyperkalemia w/IV Ca (protect heart), glucose, insulin, bicarb, albuterol, hyperventilation, kayexelate, HD.

Hyperkalemia pnuemonic: CC BIG K, (recheck K, Ca, Bicarb, Insulin, Glu, Kayexelate)

Tx hypermagnesemia (sedation, weakness) with CaCl IV and IVF.

Spironolactone (aldosterone antagonist) & propranolol (inhibits cellular K uptake) can cause hyperkalemia.

If peds hypokalemic, don't give K+ until urine output present post op.

Acute hypocalcemia shows Chvostek's (face spasm) or Trosseau's (carpal spasm) sign.

Hypocalcemia (ie parathyroids inadvertently removed) sx's occur 24-72 hrs later (laryngospasm).

Hypocalcemia can be caused by citrate (pRBC preservative) intoxication in massive transfusions.

Hypocalcemia – hypotension, flat t-waves, long QT, narrow pulse pressure, ↑ d CVP.

Citrate intoxication more likely to occur from FFP than pRBCs b/c faster administration.

Fluoride and Lithium make kidney unresponsive to ADH (nephrogenic DI).

Total Body deficit mEq of HCO3 = ECF vol (ie 0.2xkg adult & 0.4xkg neonate) multiplied by deviation of HCO3 from 24

EKG hyperkalemia: PR markedly prolonged, QRS broadened, ST elevated, and T-waves peaked.

EKG hypokalemia: PR & QT prolonged, ST depressed, T wave flat, & maybe U-wave present.

EKG hypercalcemia: prolonged PR, widened QRS, short QT interval.

EKG hypocalcemia: prolonged QT interval

EKG hypomagnesemia: prolonged QT interval

17. Pathophysiology and Anesthesia: Obstetrics

Physio CVΔs- ↑'d 45% plasma vol, 20% RBC vol, dilutional anemia, proteinuria, but ↑'d coag factors.

Physio CVΔs- CO ↑'s from 10-40% from 10th wk to 3rd trimester. After delivery ↑'d 80%. wnl 2wks post partum.

Physio CVΔs- SBP ↓'s 15%, MAP only slightly. Venous capacitance ↑'s. No Δ CVP.

Aortocaval comprsn (supine hypoTN) tx w/uterine displacement. Regional blocks compensatory responses.

When supine the blood returns via paravertebral plexuses to azygous to heart.

Physio Pulm Δs- upper airway capillary engorgement, short fat neck, use 6.5 ETT.

Physio Pulm Δs- MV ↑'d 50%, Vt >> RR, PaCO2 from 40->32. Due to ↑'d progesterone.

Physio Pulm Δs- Lung vol 20% ↓ in FRC. VC unchanged -> speeds inhalation induction.

Physio Pulm Δs- Art O2 early gestation >100mmHg, ↑d met rate & ↓FRC causes rapid ↓SaO2 on induction.

Other Δs- CNS - ↓ MAC, ↓ CSF vol, ↑'d spread in epidural space, sensitivity to LAs (peripheral nerves).

Other Δs- Renal - ↑'d RBF & GFR 50-60%. BUN/Cr upper limits of normal (50%) & ratio are ↓'d.

Other Δs- Hepatic - ↓'d albumin & psuedocholinesterase. ↑'d concentration of coagulation factors & fibrinogen.

Other Δs- GI – delayed emptying, ↓ motility (progesterone). Placental gastrin ↓'s pH of gastric contents.

GE jxn angle Δs cause ↓ LES tone. Give bicitra. H2 blockers don't ↓ acidity of present contents.

Placenta releases gastrin, lowering stomach pH. Always consider full stomach.

MOM -> 2 uterine arts/many veins -> PLACENTA -> umbilical art x2/vein x1 -> BABY (draw picture!!)

The one umbilical vein carries nutrient rich (no waste) blood from the placenta to baby.

Though liver immature will still metabolize most drugs. 75% of umbilical vein blood goes to fetal liver (protective).

Drug of choice is ephedrine based on sheep studies. Neo equally effective (newer studies). UBF not autoregulated.

Maternal systemic opioids can cause neonatal neurobehavioral changes.

Partial pressure O2 which 50% Hb is bound is 20 neonates; 27 in adults. Parturient is 30 (due to resp alkalosis).

Fetal temp warmer & 0.1 pH lower -> results in ion trapping (lido) & Bohr shift R helping w/neonatal p50 of 20.

NMBDs do not cross placenta in significant amounts. Barbs, benzos, local, opioids do. Think of BBB (corollary).

The more acidemic the fetus is, the more chance for ion trapping.

Stage 1 (0-10cm dilation) labor pain T10-L2: Somatic/visceral, uterus/cervix. Inf, mid, sup hypogastric plexuses.

Stage 2 (10cm to baby exit) labor pain S2-S4: Vaginal/peroneal. Pudendal nerves.

LEA, SAB, CSE, lumbar symp blocks (stage 1), paracervical blocks (stage 1), & pudendal (stage 2) are used.

Paracervical blocks rarely performed due to bupiv toxicity & fetal bradycardia.

Nalbuphine (2.5-5mg IV onset 30 min) is an opiate ag/antag that treats pruritis. Then use benadryl.

Metoclopramide can cause anxiety and sense of dread.

Versed & Ativan equal in fetus within minutes. Ativan can remain for wks due to inability to excrete metabolites.

Ketamine can be given to augment labor & for episiotomy repair. Use small doses totaling < 1mg/kg.

Mild overdoses of LAs in fetus manifest as hypotonicity after birth (similar to Mg toxicity (resp depression).

Altered progress of labor occurs via motor blockade, only affecting stage 2 of labor.

NO2 50% inhaled causes no loss of consciousness & no effects on labor, but often inadequate pain relief.

Absolute contraindications to neuraxial: refusal, infxn at site, coagulopathy, sepsis, bacteremia, shock.

Relative contraindications to neuraxial are ↑ ICP, multiple sclerosis (SAB), & neuromuscular disease.

HIV is not contraindication for neuraxial or blood patch.

Max Local: Lido w/o epi 5mg/kg; Lido w/epi 7mg/kg. Bupiv 2.5mg/kg. Ropiv 2mg/kg.

Alternate Max Local: Lido 300mg; Bupiv 250mg. Ropiv 200mg.

Failed DL 8x higher in OB pts: large breasts, pharyngolaryngeal edema, ↓ FRC, ↑ O2 consumption, short neck.

Pre-O2 w/3-5min 100% or 8 maximal breaths in 60 secs. LMA, fastrack available. If TTJV use 1:1 I/E ratio.

Propofol assoc'd w/maternal brady (w/sux). Reason STP used to be preferred.

VAs in excess for long periods can depress neonate, but rapidly wears off with ventilation.

Neuraxial anes shown to block stress response, ↓ EBL, ↓ postop thrombotic events, & ↓ M&M in high risk pts.

Spine has 33 vertebrae 7c, 12t, 5l, 5s, 5c. We have 31 pairs of spinal nerves.

Neuraxial approaches are midline & paramedian. Taylor approach is paramedian at L5-S1 space. Caudal is S5.

Spinal lidocaine (70mg) onset 1-3min, peak height reached 10-15 min, duration 45-75 minutes.

Spinal bupivicaine (8-12mg) onset 2-4min, peak height reached 20 min, duration 120-180 minutes.

Spinal morphine(100-200mcg) onset is 45 minutes and can last up to 24hrs.

Preservative free Chloroprocaine safe for spinal (if not then can get adhesive arachnoiditis).

Lidocaine spinal implicated in cauda equina, TNS, TRI. (Barash).

Epidural 3% Chloroprocaine (15-25mL) onset 5-10min, duration 45 minutes.

Epidural 2% Lidocaine (15-25mL) onset 10-20min, duration 60 minutes.

Epidural 0.5% Ropivicaine (15-25mL) onset 20-25min, duration 120 minutes.

Per dermatome epidural spread: Lumbar 1.5mL, Thoracic 1.0mL, Cervical 0.5mL.

Can give 10-12mL of 3% chloroprocaine epidurally for instrumental deliveries.

The more lipid soluble the LA (etidocaine/bupivicaine) the less epinephrine works.

Bupivicaine 0.75% is contraindicated in epidural space (CV toxicity due to large volume/dose req).

NaHCO3 speeds onset of epidural analgesia by 1 minute. ↓ s pH, ↑ ing unionized (active) fraction.

CSE carries risk for fetal bradycardia. Usual dose is 1mL of 0.25% isobaric Bupivicaine.

Persistent occiput posterior fetal position causes back labor (baby on back = maternal back pain).

NTG 50-150mcg IV relaxes hypetonic uterus during breech or for delivery of 2nd twin.

HELLP is severe form of pre-eclampsia. Complcxns: cerebral hemorrhage, CHF, MI, coagulopathy, seizures.

Pre-E tx is Mg (therapeutic serum 4-6 mEq/L). Mg: weakness, hypoventilation, cardiac arrest. Poteniates NMBDs.

Methylergonovine (ergots) used for atony can precipitate HTN crisis in pts with Pre-E.

EBL is 500 for SVD, 1000 for c/s, 2-5L for placenta previa/accreta/pancreta/abruptio.

If placenta previa patient is bleeding then DIC isn't triggered because loss is external.

AFE (amniotic fluid embolus) has resp distress, hypotension, & hypoxemia. Definative dx is via pathology.

Organogenesis (2-8wks), umbilical vein pH 7.35, CO2 38, PaO2 30. Maternal ↑ d FiO2 does NOT ↑ ROP.

MG babies need therapy for 3-4 wks (residual maternal IgG present). MG doesn't affect cardiac or smooth muscle.

Homozygous atypical psuedocholinesterase can still break down chloroprocaine in 2 minutes!

Mg sulfate (hypotonia/resp depression) sedation via NMDA antagonist. NOT analgesic, does NOT cause ARF.

Indomethacin is used as a tocolytic (relaxes smooth muscle). Keeps PDA open after birth.

Leading cause of maternal death is hemorrhage or hypertensive crisis depending on source.

Remember VEAL : CHOP. Fetal scalp pH near 7.0 leads to depressed neonate.

APGAR of 10 rare bc acrocyanosis persists well past 5 minutes.

Rapid IV HCO3 can cause ICH bc of rapid ↑ s in CBF. THAM (tromethamine) ↓ 's PCO2.

Infant resus: Epi dose for asytole is 20mcg/kg. Umbilical A-line optimal but technically difficult.

Infant resus: Naloxone (100mcg/kg) is contraindicated in newborns of opiate addicted mothers.

Infant resus: Use the ETT to suction after meconium aspiration (enables large particulate matter retrieval).

Prolonged LEA (>5hrs) can increase maternal core temp up to 38 degrees. Mechanism unknown.

Plica medianis dorsalis (vertical band within epidural space) is not clinically significant.

TNS is sensory ONLY pain/dysesthesia legs, buttocks. Range is 3 -14 days, but some sources say up to 6 mos.

TNS (1-4days avg) is more likely lidocaine spinal & lithotomy position and less likely in pregnancy.

TNS lat fem q nerve (most common), obturator, lumbosacral trunk (foot drop), femoral (hip flexors).

CES (diffuse axonal injury) may be spectrum w/TNS but NOT on boards. Pain, motor, bowel/bladder dysfxn.

PDPH (1% incidence). Treat with IV analgesia, caffeine (over 1-2hrs), supine postion, or EBP.

PDPH happens 50% after wet tap. Up to 25% after spinal. We likely have less % due to obesity in our region.

Spinal hematoma occurs in 1:150,000. Most use plt count of at least 80-100. See ASRA guidelines.

Early sign of total spinal is nausea (cerebral ischemia). Tx is ABCs, head down, IVF, pressors (epi 0.1-.5).

Multiple sclerosis exacerbated by SAB!!! NOT LEA or PNBs.

18. Pathophysiology and Anesthesia: Congenital/Idiopathic & Pediatrics

Congenital/Idiopathic

Acromegaly: ↑ d airway soft tissue, long mandible, neuropathy, DM, thick skin, large tongue.

Acromegaly: Test for ulnar circulation (poor in this dz) prior to radial a-line.

Beckwith Wiedeman have large tongue, omphalocele, hypoglycemia, macrosomia, polycythemia.

CDH: medical manage first! Watch for pneumo on right. RSI then decompress stomach.

Central Core Disease: Auto dominant NMD, association with MH bc defect in ryanodine receptor.

DiGeorge Syndrome (thymic hypoplasia): Hypocalcemia, micrognathia, neonatal tetany, vascular abn (TOF).

Duchenne: watch for MH, subclinical usually noticed by age 8.

Gastroschisis, no sac, to right of umbilicus. NOT associated w/cardiac defects (always a distractor).

IHSS: Minimize obstruction via ↑ preload & afterload, ↓ contractility. BBs are cornerstone of management.

IHSS: Remember SAD. Syncope, angina, & dyspnea. CHF and mitral regurgitation common.

King-Denborough: mental retardation, web neck, short stature, kyphoscoliosis, low ears, winged scapulae.

MEN2a med thyroid Ca & hyperparathyroidism. MEN2b pheo, medullary thyroid Ca, & neuromas.

MH : autosomal dominant with variable penetrance.

MH Associated with: King Denborough, Duchenne, Central Core Dz, & Osteogenesis Imperfecta.

Myelomeningocele (latex allergy) usually have Arnold-Chiari & need surg within 24 hrs after birth.

NEC due to decr mesenteric blood flow. Tx non-op unless perforation, give products early, keep sats 90-95%.

Omphalocele within sac of umbilical ring (keep PaO2 50-70mmHg). Association with cardiac defects.

Pyloric stenosis (1/500 births) med emergency. WM, 1st borns, 6wks. Sonography for dx. HypoK/Cl alk or acidosis.

TEF type C most common (eso atresia w/lower segment connected to trachea). Know VACTERL.

Tough DL: Trisomy 21, abnormal facies (Treacher, Goldenhar, Pierre-Robin), dwarfism (micrognathia).

VHL associated with hemangiomas of CNS and pheo. Stanozolol is one tx of hemangiomas.

Pediatrics

1. TBW in adults is 60% x kg. Term neonates is 80% x kg. Plasma vol (5% x kg) constant throughout life.

2. Newbord glucose 40-60 and K 4-6. Tongue and occiput large. Epiglottis large, short, & narrow.

3. Newborn larynx is C3/4 (adult C5/6), vertical vocal cords, trachea smallest at cricoid.

4. Alveoli 20 million at birth and 300 million at 18 months. Basically lungs not mature at birth.

5. FRC neonate is 25mL/kg vs adult 40mL/kg. However, FRC/TLC ratio is normal bc TLC is lower in neonate.

6. VC is 35mL/kg in infant but 70mL/kg in adult (ie adult IC is ~ 2500!).

7. Newborns have compliant rib cages, inefficient (flat) diaphragms, and premies have decr'd surfactant.

8. Hypoxia/acidosis in newborn causes persistent fetal circulation. Treat with indomethacin.

9. Normal acidosis of newborn due to renal immaturity (HCO3 & glucose loss).

10. Cardiac output is HR dependent. GFR decr'd until 1-2 yrs old.

11. Newborn Hb is 20g/dL, premie 15g/dL. HbF decreases until 6 mos old (Hb 10). P50 20 at birth.

12. Resp & CV instability can benefit from Hb >15. Immature liver (2,7,9,10). Preop FFP, pRBCs, plts available.

13. NEC due to decr mesenteric blood flow. Tx non-op unless perforation, give products early, keep sats 90-95%.

14. Omphalocele within sac of umbilical ring (keep PaO2 50-70mmHg). Association with cardiac defects.

15. Gastroschisis, no sac, to right of umbilicus. NOT associated w/cardiac defects (always a distractor).

16. TEF type C most common (eso atresia w/lower segment connected to trachea). Know VACTERL.

17. CDH, medical manage first! Watch for pneumo on right. RSI then decompress stomach.

18. Myelomeningocele (latex allergy) usually have Arnold-Chiari and need surg within 24 hrs after birth.

19. PS is medical (not surg) emergency. WM 1st borns, 6wks. Sonography used for dx. HypoK/Cl alk or acidosis.

20. URI 2-6 wks prior (0-6yrs old) may delay elective GETA. Okay to proceed with mask ventilation anesthesia.

21. Admit for observation (apnea risk) infants <60 wks PCA. UMC policy is ex-premie < 54wks PCA.

22. Preterm at risk for ROP until 44wks PCA. Keep PaO_2 70mmHg, sats 93-95% if feasible.

23. Premature (lay term) = prior to 37wks post conception & classically weighing 500-2499g at birth.

24. Preterm = infant born before 37wks (eg. 36 & 6 days). LBW is <2500g and VLBW is <1500. ELBW is <1000.

25. Usually bradycardic response to hypoxemia (in peds) precedes desaturation. Bag mask newborns (not atropine).

26. Pyloric stenosis associated with post op CNS ventilatory depression bc of CSF alkalosis.

27. Omphalocele related to cardiac problems (gastroschisis is not).

28. If peds hypokalemic, don't give K+ until urine output present post op.

29. At risk for ROP (from high FiO_2) up to 44wks PCA, and for post op apnea up to 60 wks PCA.

30. Optic ischemic injury is reason not to prolong PEDs spine surgeries >5 hrs.

31. Rib notching is seen in coarctation of the aorta.

32. First sign of total spinal in an infant (ie oops caudal) is apnea....not bradycardia (that will be distracter).

33. According to literature warming blankets most impt for pts <10kg. Then forced air warmers.

Lung Stages: embryonic/psuedoglandular/canalicular; 24wks-Birth:Saccular; Birth-3yo:Alveolar (50-500million) Peds lungs almost fully fxn'l in several hours. Common for episodes of central apnea >5 sec. Newborns have *Hering-Breuer* reflex = lung inflation leads to resp depression. Ribs more parallel, chest wall more compliant, flat diaphram w/less type 1 fibers. O_2 consumption 6mL/kg/min vs 3mL/kg/min in adults

> *Boards*** – FRC is estimated to be the same, they desat bc MVent/FRC ratio incr'd

Fetal Circulation – Placenta = fetal respiration. HbF ->fetus has incr'd temp and decrd pH to compensate for left Bohr shift; Placenta – 2art/1vein(PaO_2 35) -> 50% bypasses liver via ductus venosis to IVC ->to RA/RV (O_2 preferably thru FO to LA/LV)-> thru ductus arteriosis-> aorta -> to mother thru 2 arts 28).

> *Boards*** – fetal carotids' PaO_2 is 28.

Heart muscle immature, decr'd contractility, CHF easy. CO and end organ perf primarily = HR. Parasymp – fully fxn'l, while symp not = reason for minor stimuli causing brady in <6mos age

Newborn CO = 350ml/kg/min; 2 mo CO = 150; and Adult CO 75; Birth Hb = 19g/dL w/70% HbF, @8wks Hb is 10, HbA and 2,3DPG incr. Coags decreased at birth, but normalize in 1st yr.

Birth Cardiopulmonary Changes - Clamping cord incr's SVR, PVR decr's with (-) intrathoracic pressure; PaO_2 incr, $PaCO_2$ decr leading to reversal of fetal acidosis, ABG normal w/in 24hrs; LA pressure incr, *ductus arteriosis*->closes bc of pH and PaO_2 incr & no placental prosta-E2

Persistent Pulm HTN of Newborn (PPHN) – used to be called PFC; Causes include resp distress synd, meconium asp, hypothermia, & congenital H Dz.; Tx-aggr correction of underlying d/o. correct hypoxemia, hypercarbia, & acidosis (poss inh NO)

Renal – GFR 25% of adult value @ birth (until 1yr); Urine concentrating ability decr'd until 4 mo

Neuro – Ant fontanelle closed by 18months, post by 3 months old;

CMRO2 > child > adult > newborns/infants; Autoregulation in infants MAP 20-80 (extrapolated)

Developental Pharmacology – Pharmacokinetics/dynamics altered in early life by:

1. Vd increased – large bolus of H2O soluble med (ie NMBD) needed, but have longer t1/2

2. Protein Binding – alb (mildly low) binds weak acids, AAG (very low) binds weak bases (LA's).

3. Metabolism – generally incr'd due to incr hep blood flow, but neonates decr'd bc low cp450

4. Exc/Elimination – GFR decr'd as above, but more rapid clearance due to incr hep blood flow

IV Anesthetics – neonates possibly more sensitive to IV anesthetics because of immature BBB

Inhalational – ↑d MVent/FRC ratio -> fast CNS onset; ↑d CO slows inhalational induction; ↓d muscle/fat causes quicker equilibration of anesthetic; MAC increases with age up to 6 months then gradually decreases.

Resp Distress Syndrome – Premies are born w/ ↓'d Type 2 Pneumocytes. Surf production usually complete by 36th wk. RSD formerly termed HMD. ↑risk of RSD: asphyxia, maternal DM, mult pregnancies, C-section, cold stress. ABG: acidosis w/hypercarbia & hypoxemia. Goals are to give surfactant & keep PaO2 from 50-70mmHg & PaCO2 45-60. Can use HFJV or oscillating ventilation. Intra-op give PEEP and RR 30-50. Avoid high FiO2.

Apnea of Prematurity – apnea defined as absence of breaths for 20+ sec; less is accompanied by bradycardia. AoP usually resolves by 52nd PC week. Can be obstructive & central. Use tactile stim, O2, PPV, caffeine, monitoring.

PDA: L ->R shunting. Associated w/IVH, NEC, oliguria, & pulm dz. SBE px for 6 mos after artificial closure.

Anemia of Prematurity: ↓ epo, rbc production, lifespan, & ↑ blood draws. Most agree for Hb level of 10 for surg.

IVH – almost exclusively in premies because of spont bleeding of fragile vessels in subependymal germinal matrix around lateral ventricles. Can induce it w/awake intubations & rapid infusion of bicarb.

Retinopathy of Prematurity – formerly retrolental fibroplasias, retinal vessels vasoconstrict for maturation. Can be caused by prolonged O2 but also has happened in cyanotic infants. Sats should be maintained low to mid 90s.

Hypoglycemia – glucose crosses placenta but insulin doesn't. ↓ the maintenance by 50% bc surg ↑ glu. check qhr.

BPD: sequelae of RDS. Tachypnea, bronchospasm, O2 req, & CO2 retention. Mild, mod, or severe. Tx w/theophylline, caffeine, inhaled B2s. Anxiolysis prevent BPD spasm, avoid ETT (deep ext), LMA or regional.

Laryngeal & Tracheal Injury – subglottic stenosis common (15%) after neonatal prolonged ETT. Use smaller ETT w/air leak <30cmH2O. Tracheobronchomalacia up to 50% incidence in CLDI; due to frequent suctioning, lower airway granulomas, etc.

Post-op Apnea – formerly premature infants have apneic spells following GA. No report of post op apnea at >60 wks PCA. Prevent by using regional, IV caffeine 10mg/kg, & short acting anesthetics. Regional shown to **decrease** incidence of PoA, but 24 hr monitoring still recommended if former premie <60 wks PCA.

Normal IVF – deficit/maint/fluid loss. Use 4:2:1 if >2 wks old. If <2wks can't excrete free water so require less.

1. Calories 0-10kg = 100 kcal/kg, 11-20kg = 1000 + 50/kg over 10, 20-70kg = 1500 + 20/kg over 20

2. Fluid if <2wks 750-1000 grams AND 1-7 days old OR >1000g AND >3 days old give 125mL/kg/24hrs.

3. For every 1000 kcal expended 1000mL of water is required.

4. Use isotonic, LR preferred but NS if large volume replacement is needed. LR=130Na, 4K, 3Ca, 109Cl, 28Lac

5. Deficit is 4:2:1 x hrs fasting -> give 50% first hr, 25% each of next two hrs. If short procedure give 4mL/kg

6. Some add glucose to IVF for infants if <10kg -> usually 2% solution.

7. Fluid losses are due to evaporative, 3rd spacing, and blood loss. Use crystalloid with end pts = BP, HR, and UOP

8. Can give albumin 5-20mL/kg. If you give too much pt can get hypernatremia.

Blood

1. pRBCs -> give for Hb <7, Hb<8 if symptomatic, acute blood loss with hypovolemia, & if Hct <40% in pulm dz.

2. EBV is 95, 85, 75, 70mL/kg for premie, newborn, >3mos, and >1yr respectively. Calculate MABL.

3. Massive transfusion defined as 1 or + blood vol. Cplcxns: dilution, DIC, decr temp, pH, Ca, incr K, glu, volume

FFP

1. Used for bleeding secondary to documented coag factor deficiency or presumed from massive transfusions.

2. Calc the dose by estimating the plasma volume: TBVx(1-Hct) then multiply by 25% (factor level needed)

3. Rapid administration will cause transient hypocalcemia and decr BP. It may transmit pathogens.

Platelets

1. Indications are <50k OR <100k in presence of active bleeding. Give premature if <100 bc risk of ICH

2. Approx 5-10mL/kg should raise plt count 50-100k. In adults 1 unit incrs by 5-10k. That's why we give 6 pack.

Peds Pharmacokinetic Considerations

1. Reduced protein binding in neonates due to decr'd alb & AAG levels, also poor alb that binds less effectively.

2. Have incr'd FFAs, bilirubin, plasma acidity, metabolic activity (6-8mL/kg/min O2 consumption), body water % (Vd), CO % going to brain, and an immature BBB leading to possibly incr'd conc in CNS.

3. From age 2-6 liver has greater metabolic capacity so may require higher doses, etc of analgesics.

4. Immature renal/hepatic system in newborns may significantly alter half-lives, etc.

Peds pain meds - ASA, Tylenol, & NSAIDS used for mild-mod pain, don't cause resp depression, sedation, or dependance. Act via COX inh - AA to prosta's/thromboxane. Bronchoconstrict from shunting of AA to leukotrienes.

2. ASA rarely used bc of Reye's. Tylenol is antipyretic and poor COX inhibitor so likely central COX importance. COX 2 specific not well studied in children. Common NSAIDS used are ibuprofen, ketorolac, and naproxen.

3. Some studies show ibuprofen superior analgesic to Tylenol, but others show no difference.

4. Tramadol - Close in structure to codeine, but has 10th the affinity for μ rec, 10-15x less potent than morphine.

5. Tramadol - At normal PO doses doesn't cause resp dep, sed, or constipation. Not FDA approved in PEDS pts.

6. Ketamine - PCP derivative. Analgesic at subanesthetic doeses not revsd by naloxone. Works via NMDA and sigma opiate rec. Given any route, PO bioavailability is 25%. IV 0.5mg/kg good analgesia for 10-15 min.

7. Ketamine - Is a negative inotrope, but symp outflow offsets effect. Can ↑ ICP & hallucinations. Give benzo.

Peds Opioids

1. Opiates bind to CNS pre&post synaptic cell membranes.

2. Mu rec are found in the cortex, thalamus, periaquaductal gray, and the substantia gelatinosa of spinal cord.

3. Used in children for cough suppression and diarrhea as well as analgesia.

4. Metabolism/excretion slowed in newborns and more free fraction is less plasma alb and AAG.

5. Morphine is the prototype to which all others compared. Produce M3G and M6G. M3G-not active.

6. Fentanyl is more potent (100x); rapid on and offset; often given intranasally and via lollipop.

7. Hydromorphone is 10x more lipophillic than morphine and 5x more potent.

8. Meperidine mainly used as 1 time dose for pain, and for shivering, Normep causes seizures.

9. Methadone has the longest t1/2 (13-100+ hrs) and additionally is an NMDA antagonist.

10. Codeine is broken down to morphine (10-15%) for action. Some people lack the enzyme.

11. Oxycodone is 1st line PO opioid analgesic in children. Works in 25 minutes and lasts 4.5 hrs.

12. Nalbuphine is mu antag and k agonist. Can antagonize mu mediated effects. Has dose ceiling.

13. Naloxone is mu, k, and sigma antagonist. Elimination t1/2 only 60 minutes.

19. Pain Definitions & Chronic Pain

Pain Definitions

IUPAC - Pain is an unpleasant sensory or emotional experience associated with actual or potential tissue damage or described in terms of such damage.

Addiction – uncontrollable psychological compulsion to repeat a behavior despite negative consequences.

Akasthesia – feeling of inner restlessness, uneasiness, antipsychotic meds (abilify). Suicide risk.

Allodynia: lowered threshold: stimulus and response mode differ

Allodynia: Pain due to a stimulus, which does not normally provoke pain.

Analgesia: Absence of pain in response to stimulation which would normally be painful.

Anesthesia Dolorosa - Pain in an area or region which is anesthetic. Example after a neurolytic nerve block.

Causalgia/CRPS2 - syndrome burning pain, allodynia, & hyperpathia after traumatic nerve lesion

Central Pain - Pain initiated or caused by a primary lesion or dysfunction in the central nervous system.

Dysesthesia - *unpleasant* abnormal sensation, spontaneous or evoked. It includes hyperalgesia & allodynia.

Hyperalgesia: increased response: stimulus and response mode are the same

Hyperpathia: raised threshold: stimulus and response mode may be the increased response: same or different

Hypoalgesia: raised threshold: stimulus and response mode are the same lowered response:

Hypoesthesia - Decreased sensitivity to stimulation, excluding the special senses.

Hyperalgesia - An increased response to a stimulus which is normally painful.

Hyperesthesia - ↑ d sensitivity to stimulation, light touch = pain. Includes allodynia & hyperalgesia

Hyperpathia - syndrome characterized by abnormally painful rxn to stimulus, especially a repetitive stimulus.

Hypoalgesia - Diminished pain in response to normally painful stimulus.

Malingering – to eggagerate or pretend incapacity to avoid work (secondary gain).

Neuralgia - Pain in the distribution of a nerve or nerves.

Neuritis - a special case of neuropathy and reserved for inflammatory processes affecting nerves.

Nociceptor - A receptor preferentially sensitive to a stimulus, which would become noxious if prolonged.

Noxious Stimulus – one that is damaging to normal tissues

Pain Threshold - The least experience of pain, which a subject can recognize.

Pain Tolerance Level - The greatest level of pain, which a subject is prepared to tolerate.

Neuritis - Inflammation of a nerve or nerves. Note: Not to be used unless inflammation is present.

Neurogenic Pain - initiated or caused by a primary lesion, dysfxn, or transitory perturbation in PNS or CNS

Neuropathic Pain - initiated or caused by a primary lesion or dysfunction in the nervous system.

Neuropathy - disturbance of fxn or pathological Δ in a nerve: mono, poly. Chronic, not temporary like neurogenic.

Paresthesia - An abnormal sensation, whether spontaneous or evoked. Not uncomfortable like dysesthesia.

Psuedoaddiction is incorrectly diagnosed addiction. Iatrogenic undertreatment of pain.

Tolerance – body becomes less responsive to substance or insult with repeated use or exposure.

Chronic Pain

Transduction: Noxious stimuli of PNs releases local inflammatory mediators. Block with LAs, NSAIDS, etc.

Transmission: after transduction, impulse travels A-delta & C fibers to doral horn. Block with regional.

Perception: Afferent fibers of dorsal horn travel via ST tract to reticular formation (CNS). Block w/ opiods, etc.

Modulation: Efferent pathways w/inhibitory NTs modify the afferent nociceptive information. Use many things.

Psychological: contribute to experience of pain, ie "battle" or a lion bit off your arm, but you still need to run.

Nociceptors transmit via A-delta (m) & C fibers (un-m) to dorsal horn (synapsing in SubGel/Lam 5 [WDRs]).

Wide dynamic range neurons (WDRs) cause "wind up" phenomenon.

Signals ascend via spinothalamic, reticular, and mesencephalic tracts to CNS. Modulated at many levels.

Dorsal col/medial lemniscus (touch/prop/vib) -> DR 1° -> medulla (2° decussate)-> VPL (3° to cortex).

Anterolateral col (sharp pain/temp) -> DR 1° -> 2 levels up (Lissuaer's) synapse in SubGel (2° decussate)-> VPL.

Receptors: Mu 1 rec cause prolactin release (women on heroin), Mu 2 rec = resp depression, kappa = dysphoria.

Type A alpha: myelinated; large motor, proprioception, fast conduction

Type A beta: myelinated; small motor, touch, pressure, fast conduction

Type A gamma: myelinated; muscle tone, fast conduction, motor

Type A delta: myelinated; pain, temperature, touch, fast conduction, sharp, well localized.

Type B: myelinated; sympathetic preganglionic (autonomics)

Type C: unmyelinated; dull pain, temp, touch, visceral, poorly localized; slow conduction, symp post-ganglionic

Migraines 40% bilateral, photophobia, nausea. Tx w/triptans, NSAIDs, Midrin, & dyhydroergotamine.

CRPS 1 (RSD): no discreet injury or nerve damage; allodynia, hyperagesia, dystrophic/temp Δs.

CRPS 2 (causaglia): injury to major nerve (usually 1 mos after); allodynia, hyperagesia, dystrophic/temp Δs.

Tx CRPS1 with daily stellate ganglion block, steroids, SSRIs, and TCAs.

Phantom limb pain treated by tegretol, TENS unit, epidural morphine, and calcitonin.

Phantom limb pain incidence is decreased by neuraxial analgesia for the surgery.

Fibromyalgia (need 11/18 diffuse trigger pts) non-dermatomal. Above/below diaphragm. Unknown etiology.

Tx of fibromyalgia includes amitriptyline (elavil), Lyrica (pregabalin), and Cymbalta (duloxatine).

Meralgia Paresthetica: compression of lat fem cutaneous nerve by inguinal ligament, anterolateral thigh pain/numbness.

Trigeminal neuralgia (V2) tx'd w/carbamazepine & Gasserian ganglion blockade (watch out total spinal).

Five A's of clinical opiates: activity, analgesia, affect, adverse rxns, aberrant behavior.

Do NOT use clonidine for post herpetic neuralgia. -> ineffective.

PCA used in pts >6yo. Cons are if pt unable to use or family member presses button for the pt overdosing them.

Continuous IV Opioid Infusion (CIV) is alternative to PCA for pts <7yo, MR, or cognitively impaired.

Transition from PCA, CIV, CEA, PCEA is sometimes difficult. Use conversion tables for opiates.

Use alternative meds for weaning such as PO/IV combo regimens, Tylenol, Tramadol, oxycodone.

Morphine IV/IM equivalent to 100mg Meperidine is 10mg. SEE equivalent dosages in opiate sections.

Non-drug modalities for pain include distraction, acupuncture, and TENs.

Most common side effect of long term opioid use is constipation.

Cancer pain treated with morpine, if bone pain (NSAIDS), and oral route is preferred.

Bretylium causes release of NE then inhibits further release. HTN then hypotension. Tx for CRPS1.

Bretylium – used for IV regional in RSD (CRPS1). Also IV regional = guanethidine & reserpine are used.

Right stellate controls chronotropy & dromotropy. Left controls inotropy. Know C6, temp change, tx CRPS.

Left SGB shortens QT intervals, and is a treatment for congenital long QT syndrome.

SGB: symp block of head and upper ext. Can get Horner's synd w/o upper extremity block.

SBG: Adequacy of symp block assessed by rise in temp of at least 2 degrees Celsius.

If bilateral SGB risk for bilateral RLN (all laryngeal muscles except cricothyroid) paralysis (VCs will be adducted).

RSD (chronic) has dystrophic changes in skin and bone demineralization.

Horners: ptosis, miosis, anhydrosis, hoarsness (RLN), enophthalamos, nasal stuffy (vasc engorgement), flushing.

Neurolytic block usually not used on peripheral nerves bc of denervation dysesthesias. Have to repeat q6 mos.

Alcohol (causes intense pain) is hypobaric and phenol is hyperbaric. Both are used for neurolytic blocks.

Celiac plexus (L1 level, retroperitoneal) block complications are hypotension & diarrhea (vagal overreactivity).

Inter/intrapleural catheters are most effective in children, PFTs improve.

Epidural steroid injections for chronic pain more likely to work for radicular pain (not back pain).

Ketamine has been shown to prevent hyperalgesia in perioperative period. 1mg/kg intraop and/or post op infusion.

Ketamine also been shown to prevent opioid induced hyperalgesia in chronic opiate therapy.

Ziconitide (25AA-peptide, selective N-type CCB) is a potent intrathecal analgesic for refractory chronic pain.

20. Anatomy & Regional/Acute Pain

Anatomy

Dermatomes: C4 clavicle/shoulders, C6 thumb, T2/T3 axilla, T4 nipple, T6 xyphoid, T7 lower border of scapula

Dermatomes: T10 umbilicus, L4 anterior knee, L5 bottom of foot, S1/S2 back of legs, S5 butt hole.

SLN (internal branch): thyrohyoid membrane sensation to epiglottis, vocal cords, and above area.

SLN (external branch): motor to cricothyroid muscle (tenses vocal cords). RLN abducts.

RLN sensation below the cords, motor to all laryngeal muscles except cricothyroid. If paralyzed **VCs adducted.**

Cricopharyngeus muscle (aka LES) is innervated by the vagus nerve (CNX). X also provides sensation to entire trachea.

Brachial plexus (C5-T1): 5 roots to 3 trunks (above 1st rib) to divisions to cords to terminal nerves (in axilla).

Lateral cord terminates as the musculocutaneous nerve. Medial cord -> ulnar nerve. Posterior -> radial nerve.

Femoral/obturator/lat fem cutaneous (T12-L4); Sciatic Nerve (L4-S3).

Median nerve motor supply to opponens pollicis & flexor pollicis brevis. Ulnar supplies adductor pollicis.

Testicular innervation can be traced up to the T10 dermatome level.

Nausea after neuraxial due to sympathectomy, HypoTN, & unopposed parasympathetic to GI tract.

Sacral hiatus (S4-5 interspace) is lower border of epidural space. Caudal performed at S5.

Right stellate controls chronotropy & dromotropy (conduction speed). Left controls inotropy.

SGB located at level of C6, know temp change, tx CRPS, etc.

Sympathetic trunk extends from C2 to coccyx. (24 ganglia).

RCA supplies AV node in 90% of pts. Blockage associated with inferior (lead II) ischemia & heart block.

Regional/Acute Pain

Acute pain usually denotes tissue injury, inflammation, or infection.

Colombs Law – $I = k\ (a/r^2)$: Clear motor response from 0.2-0.5 improves efficacy of stimulating for PNBs.

Retrobulbar block yields akinesis and sensory block of the globe (CN 2, 3, & 6). Misses CN 4.

Interscalene block performed at c6 level, across from cricoid cartilage, in groove, circa the EJ.

Interscalene sometimes spares ulnar nerve (T8,C1 lower trunk) & blocks phrenic in up to 100% of patients.

Axillary block can miss intercostobrachial nerve (T2 intercostal) & median cutaneous nerve (proximal biceps cuff).

Axillary block risks missing the musculocutaneous, must supplement 3-5cc lido in AC fossa (coracobrachialis).

Bier block 40mL 0.5% lido, cuff at 100mmHg above SBP, minimum 30min tourniquet time, max 2 hrs.

Median nerve block at elbow is 3-5mL just medial to brachial artery or line connecting med & lat epicondyles.

Median nerve blocked at elbow just medial to brachial artery. Radial is b/t brachioradialis & biceps tendon.

Ankle block must block 5 nerves. They are saphenous, sural, post tib, superficial & deep peroneal.

Deep peroneal: is motor to flexors of toes, anterior tibialis (dorsiflexion), sensory between first 2 toes.

Deep peroneal: located between ext hallicus longus & ext digitorum longus tendons on anterior ankle.

Superficial peroneal: is foot eversion and sensory to top of foot (excluding great toe web space).

Sural nerve is sensory (only) to the lateral malleolus, Achilles tendon, ankle joint, and 5th toe.

Saphenous nerve: terminal sensory (only) branch of femoral. The vein & nerve are just anterior to medial malleolus.

Posterior tibial nerve: location posterior aspect of medial malleolus.

Neither saphenous nor sural nerves contain motor fibers.

Intercostal blocks (rib fx's) 8-10cm from spine to avoid missing lateral cutaneous branches. VAN, nerve most inferior.

Cauda equina syndrome associated with maldistribution of LA within intrathecal space.

Differential nerve blockade related to density is sympathetic, pain, proprioception, then motor.

LA speed of onset related to pKa & conc. Potency related to lipid solubility.

Greatest plasma concentration post block: intercostal > caudal (gavity) > epidural > brachial plexus > fem/sciatic.

Intercostobrachial nerve innervates posterior medial arm. Musculocutaneous anterolateral forearm.

T1-T4 are cardiac accelerator fibers and would not affect DM autonomic neuropathy if blocked.

Procaine NOT effective as a topical agent. EMLA has lidocaine and prilocaine (takes 30-60min to work).

Etidocaine and bupivicaine are NOT prolonged w/use of vasopressors in neuraxial anesthesia.

To make solution hyperbaric add glucose, hypobaric (add sterile water), isobaric (add CSF).

21. Acid-Base & ABG

1. Alkalosis: dysrhythmias, coronary vasoconstriction, decr Ca & K, incr R -> L shunt, L shift (tissue hypoxia)

2. Acidosis: dysrhythmias, Incr PVR and ICP, incr K. Incr's Ca until severe acidosis.

3. Mixed venous O2 sat increased by sepsis, cyanide tox, incr'd CO, incr'd Hb, dyshemoglobinemias

4. OxyHb Curve to R: H+, incr 2,3 DPG, HbSS, Hbthal, VA's, pregnancy, ↑ d CO2, hyperthermia.

5. OxyHb Curve to L: OH-, decr 2,3 DPG, pRBC transfusion, ↓ CO2, hypothermia, metHb, COHb.

6. ABG alpha stat: relies on temperature uncorrected ABG values. Most common (we use).

7. ABG pH stat: Give systemic CO2 to keep pH 7.4 & PCO2 40. Attempts to correct for temp/partial pressure error.

8. Normal anion gap is 5-12mEq/L. If > 12 etiology MUDPILES. If normal = diarrhea, acetazolamide, fistulas, etc.

9. Anion Gap: MUDPILES: methanol, uremia, DKA, paraldehyde, isoniazid, lactate, ethylene glycol, salicylates

10. Normal Gap: BADR: Bicarbonate loss (diarrhea), acid loads, dilution of HCO3 by normal saline, renal defects.

11. Acute inc of PaCOs 10mmHg will decr pH 0.08 units; HCO3 decr's 5 mEq/L each 10mm decr of PaCO2 <40.

12. For every 0.08 change in pH there is an inverse change in K of 0.5mEq/L.

13. Most impt buffer system is bicarbarbonate. Others are phosphate, protein, & hemoglobin systems.

14. At birth umbilical artery has lower PaO2 (20) then vein (30). PaCO2 50 & 40 respectively.

15. At 60 min the newborn PaO2 is 60mmHg, @24hrs it is 70, then trends towards 100 (adult value).

16. Co-oximetry measures abnormal Hb species, Met, CO, sulfHb.

17. Measured PaO2 (falsely low) decr's by 6% per Celsius below 37. Because of dissolved O2.

18. With chronic A/B abnormalities, oxyHb curve resets due to altered metabolism of 2,3 DPG.

19. Total Body deficit mEq of HCO3 = ECF vol (ie 0.2xkg) multiplied by deviation of HCO3 from 24

20. ABG: pH measurement relies on Sanz electrode, PCO2 on Severinghaus electrode, & PO2 on Clark electrode.

21. Reason for ↓ d EtCO2 in ↓ d CO/trauma is V/Q = infinity. Vent but no perfusion (no gas exchange). Huge A-a!

22. Metabolic alkalosis caused by vomiting, nasogastric suctioning, thiazide & loop diuretics.

23. HCO3 can cause IVH, hypernatremia, hyperosmolarity, & left Bohr shift (alkalosis).

24. PO2 & PCO2 values in hyperthermic pt will be artificially elevated. More heat = more dissolved in solution.

22. Preoperative Concerns

As a general rule, most medications can be continued up until the time of surgery

ASA: 2:mild dz (no limitations), 3:severe (limitations), 4:(incapacitating), 5:(24hrs before death), 6:brain dead.

NPO guidelines: clears 2hrs, breast milk 4 hrs, non-human milk/light snack 6hrs, fried/fatty/large/meat 8hrs.

Delay Electives: MI within 6 months, new unstable cardiac rhythm, severe coagulopathy, unclear hypoxia.

Ascertain "true" allergic rxns vs unusual, unexpected, or unpleasant reactions to medications.

True allery: skin manifestations, facial/oral swelling, SOB, choking/wheezing, or vascular collapse.

Hx of shellfish or seafood allergy has NOT been linked to allergy to IV iodine contrast.

Newer Alzheimers meds (donezepil, galantamine, rivastigmine) can prolong sux action.

Stopping smoking 6-8wks may ↓ airway hyperreactivity, post-op pulm complcxns, & wound infxn.

Stopping smoking 12 hours may reduce nicotine & HbCO levels promoting better tissue oxygenation.

Stimulant use will cause altered metabolism and/or effect of meds. (ie ephedrine in meth addicts).

Recent hx (2wks) of URI in peds ↑ s chance of bronch/laryngospasm during induction/emergence.

Pts w/DM may be difficult intubations due to TMJ/cerivical arthritis (due to synovial glycosylation).

Untreated HTN leads to BP lability intraop as well as relative hypovolemia.

Acute stimulants (meth/cocaine) ↑ MAC, acute downers (EtOH, benzos) ↓ MAC. And visa versa.

RSI/awake intubation if hiatal hernia, pregnant, GERD symptoms, full stomach, trauma, gastroparesis.

Airway exam: TM distance, mouth opening, jaw protrusion, Mallampati, cervical ROM, dention.

Tough DL: cerival disk dz, infxns, tumors, obese, trauma, radiation/burns, acromegaly, scleroderma.

Tough DL: Trisomy 21, abnormal facies (Treacher, Goldenhar, Pierre-Robin), dwarfism (micrognathia).

Nasotracheal intubation contraindicated: coagulopathy, facial fxs (Lefort is tested).

PFTs normal: TLC 5.5L, VC 4L, FRC 2.5L, RV 1.5L, FEV1 3.2L (0.8 of VC).

PFTs: Obstructive pattern if lung volumes ↑ d TLC, FRC, RV & FEV1 <80%.

PFTs: Restrictive pattern if lung volumes ↓ d with normal or ↑ d FEV1/FVC ratio.

PFTs rarely indicated: lung or tracheal resection, etc.

Murmurs (diastolic almost always pathologic) may need cardiology consultation.

Order chemistry based on H&P. Pt on diuretics, digoxin, aminoglycocides.

Order CBC/coags if bleeding anticipated, anticoagulation planned.

Order EKG if risk factors for CAD (HTN, DM, smoker, etc); or if M>45 & F>55.

Order CXR only when clinically indicated (malignancy, heavy smoker, elderly w/pulm symptoms, etc).

If BP not within 20% of baseline or DBP >115, elective surg needs to be postponed.

Perioperative longacting BB (metoprolol) therapy has been shown to ↓ myocardial ischemic episodes.

Hold ACE-I day of surgery: can lead to unresponsive hypotension on induction.

Hold metformin: ↑ s insulin sensitivity, assoc'd w/lactic acidoisis in pts w/CHF, renal failure, shock, etc.

Metformin: biguanide (lactic acidosis) & should hold 48 hrs prior to surgery, newer data 24hrs.

Can procede w/asymptomatic hypokalemia >2.7. Tx hyperkalemia if >6 and EKG changes.

Can pretreat asthma pts with duonebs. FSG on all DM. Usually tx w/insulin if >200.

Pulm asp: pretreat with H2 blockers (ranitidine, famotidine). PPIs too slow so must take PM prior.

Pulm asp: bicitra (30mL works for 30 min), reglan (speeds gastric emptying) can cause dystonia (give slowly).

Antiemetics: zofran, droperidol, haldol, decadron, phenergan, reglan, scopolamine, benadryl (peds).

Present risks & alternatives. Be concise, reassuring, unhurried, informative,

Risks GETA: sore throat, N/V, dental injury, MI, stroke, death (1:200k), post op ventilation.

Risks Lines: bleeding, infxn, nerve, tendon damage, hemothorax, or pneumothorax.

Risks Regional: headache, line risks, as well as GETA risks bc that is alternative after failed regional.

Risks Transfusion: fever, infectious hepatitis, HIV infxn, hemolytic reactions.

Anesthetic Plan: need for premeds, eval for invasive monitoring, anesthetic options, post-op pain control.

23. Postoperative Concerns/PACU & Critical Care

Postoperative Concerns/PACU

Hypovolemia most common cause of hypotension in PACU. Others are bleeding, osmotic polyuria, & third spacing.

Treat HTN & tachycardia by cause. Pain relief, BBs, CCBs, hydralazine, nitrates, benzos, antipsychotics, etc.

Hypoxemia: atelectasis, hypovent, diffusion (N2O), airway obstruction, bronchospasm, aspiration, PTX, PE, etc.

Naloxone 40-80 mcg IV titrated to effect. Onset 1-2min (lasts for 30-60min). Watch for re-narcotization.

Flumazenil 0.2-1mg IV over 5 min up to max of 5mg. Onset 1-2min, peak 10min, short half life (monitor closely).

Watch for wound hematoma in: thyroid, parathyroid, CEA, neck dissections, tracheal surgery (also VC paralysis).

Oliguria defined as < 0.5mL/kg/hr. Hypovolemia most common cause. Give IVF.

Pre renal: hypovolemia, ↓ d cardiac output, compartment syndrome (↓ d renal perfusion).

Intra renal: ATN due to hypoperfusion (hypvolemia again!), sepsis, toxins (myoglobin, nephrotoic meds), & trauma.

Post renal: urinary catheter obstruction, iatrogenic damage to the ureters.

Delayed awakening: most common is resid anesthesia, then metabolic (ie ↓ glu), neuro damage (hypoperfusion)

Emergence delerium: excitement alternating w/lethargy, confusion. More common in elderly, dementia, psych dz.

Awareness/recall detected in 1/1000 patients or even more frequently. Reassurance & sympathetic care.

PONV common (GETA>Regional). Tx scopolamine patch, dexamethasone, prop (10mg), zofran, phenergan.

Hypothermia: vasoconstrict (HTN), ↑ CO but hypoperfusion, impairs plts, wound infxn, lengthens stays.

Max FiO2 via nasal canula is 45% at 6L/min. Miller says max without intubation is 50% FiO2.

Common peroneal nerve most common lower extremity nerve injury from postioning. Ulnar overall.

Crossed legs during anesthesia results in Sural nerve injury, not peroneal.

Acute respiratory failure defined as PaO2<60 despite O2 support (FM) in absence of R->L intracardiac shunt.

Blocking dopamine rec (droperidol) -> can cause acute dytonia (torticollis). Tx with benadryl.

Shivering can ↑ O2 consumption up to 400%. SBP & HR ↑ -> ischemia. Tx HR before temp if ischemia.

A physician is responsible for discharge of a patient from PACU. Aldrete score or others can be used.

Phase 1 Recovery: from d/c of anesthetics until recovery of motor & protective reflexes (PACU d/c criteria).

Phase 2 Recovery: from meeting d/c criteria from PACU to ASU or floor monioting until d/c'd home.

Phase 3 Recovery: monitoring at home by a responsible adult.

PACU discharge criteria for outpt surgery do NOT include drinking water or voiding

Fast Tracking: skip phase 1 monitoring (ie do stage 1 in the OR), and go directly to phase/stage 2 (ie floor).

Fast Tracking Criteria: baseline awake, vitals & sx's unlikely to need meds, no active bleeding, sats >94% for 3min.

Most Common cause for re-admission is intractable vomiting.

Critical Care

Some intubation criteria RR> 30, PaO2 <60, sat <75, PACO2 > 50, worsening symp's, burns, CPAP failure.

Some extubation criteria Vc >15mL/kg, RR<30, PaO2>60 on FiO2 50%, A-a <350, pH >7.3, PCO2<50, HD stable

Normal Vd/Vt ratio is 0.3. If Vd/Vt ratio > 0.6 then intubation is warranted. See intubation criteria.

Status asthmaticus tx'd with IV steroids (gold std), inhaled b-agoniss, & possibly general anes.

Normal vital capacity is 70mL/kg, so ~5L is normal. Anatomic dead space is 2mL/kg (~150mL).

Respiratory quotient is CO2 produced divided by O2 consumed. Fat=1. Carbs=0.8, Protein=0.7, Normal diet=0.84

Nasal canula, venturi mask, non-rebreating, or t-piece seldom provide >50% FiO2 -> Miller.

Critical illness myopathy can occur after prolonged paralysis, especially when steroids are being used.

Use intermittent paralysis (not continuous, ie. not longer than 2 days), monitor with twitch monitor.

Brain death only applies in absence of hypothermia, hypotension, NMBDs, & other meds (sedatives).

ROP (premies) ↑ s with low birth weight & comorbidities. Correlates better with PaO2 than with PAO2.

Disadvantage of PCV is that tidal volume is not guaranteed (mandatory rate and insp time are set).

When ETT in place for 2-3wks, predisposes to subglottic stenosis -> trach patient.

The major effect of PEEP in lungs is to ↑ FRC. Avoid >20cm H2O = max tracheal capillary pressure (cuff).

In ARDS a Vt of >10ml/kg is associated with ↑ d mortality. Use lower Vt (6-8ml/kg).

Early elective tracheal intubation advised when obvious signs of heat injury to airway.

CRRT is for sicker patients who cannot tolerate hemodynamic Δs of standard intermittent dialysis.

Age >70, steroids, renal failure, burns, head trauma ↑ risk of nosocomial infxns (impaired immunity).

Intubation is single most important risk factor for developing nosocomial pneumonia.

Systemic venodilation and transudation of fluid into tissues causes relative hypovolemia in sepsis.

Abrupt TPN withdrawl can cause hypoglycemia due to ↑ d insulin levels. (give 10% glucose afterwards).

Abrupt d/c of TPN causes hypoglycemia/tachycardia. Watch for CVL change without checking placement.

24. Buzz/Keywords & Eponyms

Addison's dz is decr'd cortisol. On chronic corticosteroids, require stress dose to prevent CV collapse.

Aldrete score – used in PACU as criteria for discharge.

Bainbridge = Atrial stretch (Bainbridge reflex) resulting in increased HR. Think Frank starling mechansim

Barlow's Syndrome: mitral valve prolapse click murmur

Beck's Triad: elevated CVP, hypotension, & quiet heart sounds in cardiac tamponade

Beckwith Wiedeman: peds have large tongue, omphalocele, hypoglycemia, macrosomia, polycythemia.

Bernoulli's Principle = ↑d speed of fluid ↓s lateral pressure/force. Reason airplane wings work.

Bohr effect = the effect of PaCO2 and pH on oxyHb curve

Bohr Equation (dead space:tidal vol ratio) = Vd/Vt = (PaCO2 – PETCO2)/PaCO2, normal is <0.3

Botox mech is blocking release of AcH at cholinergic terminals. Does not affect storage, conduction, etc.

Boyle's Law = At fixed temp, volume & pressure are inversely proportional. Use P1/V1 = P2/V2 for tank questions.

Chi-square test is nonparametric stat that uses nominal (categorical) or ordinal data. Uses frequencies.

CO = SV x HR; SVR=(MAP-CVP)/CO x 80; Resistance = pressure / flow.

Cor pulmonale: RVH in response to pulm HTN. Classicly due to intrinsic pulmonary process (ie chronic HPV).

Cushing's Triad = HTN (widened pulse pressure), bradycardia, & resp irregularity due to ↑d ICP.

Daily cortisol secretion 30, minor surg 50, major surg 75-150, high stress 150-300.

Decadron offers no water retention; that's advantage over hydrocortisone and methylprednisolone.

DiGeorge (thymic hypoplasia): Hypocalcemia, micrognathia, neonatal tetany, vascular abn (TOF).

Ebsteins Anomaly: downward displacement of tricuspid valve causing RA enlargement. Associated with WPW & PFO.

Eisenmengers: R->L (hypoxic) shunt due to prior L->R shunt reversal due to ↑d right sided pressures.

Fick Equation: VO2 = CO x (CaO2 – CvO2); calculate VO2 (O2 consumption). Normal is 3.5mL/kg/min

Ficks Diffusion: Gas thru membrane directly prop to pressure, area, & inversely to thickness/molecular wt

First American Academic Anesthesiologist was Ralph Waters.

Frank-Starling = (vol/pressure) is larger preload results in incr'd CO/SV. EF normally remains same.

Frank-Starling = (vol/pressure) larger preload results in incr'd CO to match preload. EF normally remains same.

Garlic may have antineoplastic, hypolipidemic, & antiplatelet activity.

GCS 3-15, eyes (4), verbal (5), motor (6). Will get you with the middle numbers. Know them.

Grahams Law: diffusion coefficient inversely proportional to square root of molecular weight.

Hagan Pouisielle = laminar flow (velocity) thru tube; $V = [\pi r^4 \Delta P] / 8L\mu$; impt numbers are the 4 & 8.

Hagan Pouisielle also = Resistance = $(8L\mu)/ (\pi r^4)$; μ = viscosity

Haldane effect: deoxygenation of Hb ↑s ability to carry CO2. Inverse is reason COPD get ↑d PaCO2 after we ↑ FiO2.

Hampton's Hump – seen on CXR of pulmonary embolus

Henderson Hasselbalch Eq: pKa + log [Base/Acid] = 6.1 + log [HCO3/(0.03xPaCO2)]

Henry's Law: at constant temp the solubility of gas in liquid is proportional to partial pressure of the gas above the liquid.

Hering-Breuer reflex = lung inflation leads to resp depression, newborns have

Laplace's Law: balloon, less force is need to distend alveoli that are already open (atelectasis).

Methadone NMDA antag, opiate ag, long t½ 30hrs, blocks euphoric effects of other opiates, long withdrawl synd.

Meyer Overton theory is related to oil/gas partition coefficients.

Meyer-Overton theory (critical volume hypothesis) suggests membrane expansion mechanism for VAs.

Oculocardiac is V1 to CN10.

Ohm's Law = V = IR

Oncotic/Interstitial pressure equation = $Jv = Kf ([Pc - Pi] - \partial [\pi c - \pi i])$

Ondine's curse = abnormal hypoxic/hypercapnic drive is seen in NSGY pts, premies <60wks, OSA, & obesity.

Pascal's Principle: Hydraulics, pressure exerted on incompressible fluid is transmitted equally in all directions.

Pickwickian = old term for obesity related hypoventilation syndrome. Decr sat at night leads to HTN.

Pts need stress dose steroids if on prednisone >5-10mg/day, >1wk duration, within the year.

Pulsus Paradoxus defined as >10mmHg inspiratory ↓ in SBP. Due to ↑ d intrapericardial pressure. (tamponade).

Reynolds # = dimensionless # that gives ratio of inertial ($\rho V2/L$) forces over viscous ($\mu V/L2$) forces.

Subclavian steal syndrome (↓ d carotid flow due to trauma/malformations) worsened by SGB-> vasodilates arm.

Think of V=IR (Ohm's) so then R=V/I, so SVR (resistance) = pressure(voltage)/flow(current).

VHL associated with hemangiomas of CNS and pheo. Stanozolol is one tx of hemangiomas.

Wernicke-Korsakoff: seen in alcolholism thiamine deficiency -> confusion, ataxia, nystagmus

West Zones = Zone 1 develops with PP (vent but not perfused). 2&3 increase in vascular pressure. 2 is best.

WPW w/A-Fib: don't give nodal agents. Cardiovert if wide complex. Procainamide if narrow.

WPW w/SVT: vagal maneuvers, adenosine 3-12mg IV (1st line), esmolol, procainamide, cardiovert, AVOID digoxin.

WPW: delay along Kent fibers causing shortened PR, delta wave, paroxysmal atrial tachycardia, wide QRS, SVT

Zollinger Ellison Syndome: gastric acid hypersecretion, peptic ulcers, gastrinomas (in pancreas); present w/diarrhea.

25. Everytime Board Questions

LEA, SAB, CSE, lumbar symp blocks (stage 1), paracervical blocks (stage 1), & pudendal (stage 2) are used.

Mg sulfate (hypotonia/resp depression) sedation via NMDA antagonist. NOT analgesic, does NOT cause ARF.

Multiple sclerosis exacerbated by SAB!!! NOT LEA or PNBs.

Type A delta: small myelinated; sharp pain & *Type C*: unmyelinated dull pain, temp, are primary nociceptors.

At birth umbilical artery has lower PaO2 (20) then vein (30). PaCO2 50 & 40 respectively.

Only coag factor not produced in liver is factor 8 -> endothelial cells. Factor 7 is shortest t1/2 (6hrs).

One unit of platelet concentrate will raise plt count but 5-10 cells/mcL. So 6pack ~50k.

Porphyria Cutanea Tarda avoid skin pressure. Stress dehydration, fasting, infxn cause crises. STP (AIP) doesn't induce.

Blood storage time 3-5 wks with 70% RBC viability 24 hrs after transfusion. Plt storage is 5 days at 22C.

26. Random Pearls

1. Reason for $PaCO_2$ ~ CBF (within $PaCo_2$ 20-80) is CO_2 mediated alterations in perivascular pH constrict/vasodilate cerebrovascular arterioles. Incr'd $PaCo_2$ (or acidosis) dilates cerebral vessels, increasing ICP.

2. NSAIDS/ASA can shunt arachadonic acid to leukotrienes leading to bronchospasm in asthma pts.

3. Core Competencies: Prof, Interper Com, Med Knowledge, Systems Based Prac, Pt Care, Practice Based Learning

4. Hereditary angioedema (episodic airway edema) is C1 esterase inhibitor def'cy. Give stanozolol or C1INH conc.

5. Providers should always know location of nearest defibrillator, fire-extinguisher, gas shut off valves, O2, & exits.

6. Dexametomadine good for MAC cases on patients with severe pulm HTN.

7. With adult cath lab sick patients attempt spont ventilation. PPV increases pulm vasc resistance.

8. Nicardipine (non cardiac CCB) reason for use in neuro aneurysms vs NTG is (worse incr ICP with NTG?)

ABneg pts cannot safely receive Oneg plasma (FFP) due to Anti A&B antibodies in that plasma.

ABO status of platelet not as crucial as Rh status.

Above Co2 of 100mm CO_2 becomes a ventilatory depressant (CO2 narcosis).

ABX only indicated after aspiration of fecal matter or SBO. Don't lavage or use steroids.

Aortic bodies afferent limb is glossopharyngeal nerve & efferent is vagus.

Apneic threshold in humans is 5mmHg below the resting $PaCO_2$.

Can give cosyntropin for PDPH.

Cell saver is RBCs, saline, possibly some meds (heparin). No factors, plts, or calcium is salvaged.

Central response occurs rapidly (1min) after change in $PaCO_2$. Accounts for 85% or response to CO2.

Citrate is metabolized by the liver.

Cryo & FFP can be given w/o regard to Rh status bc don't contain red cells or platelets.

CXR may not show evidence of aspiration until 6-12 hrs -> in RLL.

Deadspace is ventilated but not perfused. Shunt is perfused but not ventilated.

DIC: PTT >15 sec, Fibrinogen <150 (300 if preg), plt count <150k, bleeding or thrombosis possible.

Dopamine 1-2mcg/kg/min (D1&2), 2-10mcg/kg/min Beta, >10 alpha predominates

During apnea, CO2 rises 6mmHg the 1st min, then 3mm/min every minute after.

Endobronchial intubation is NOT detected by capnography. Capnography uses infrared spectrometry.

Etomidate inhibits conversion of cholesterol to cortisol.

Fluosol-DA (20mL/kg) incr's O2 content & improves SvO2 (used for Jehovah's witnesses).

Gastric acid aspiration is at least 25mL (pH<2.5) & leads to atelectasis, pneumonitis, & ARDS.

Hallmark of cyanide toxicity is unexplained metabolic acidosis.

Hemolytic transfusion rxn can occur w/as little as 50mL blood (amt that exceeds haptoglobin binding capacity).

Heparin mechanism is an antithrombin 3 cofactor neutralizes 9/10/11 and inactivates thrombin.

Heparin t1/2 is 1 hr. Both PT and PTT are prolonged.

Hexadimethrine is anticoagulant used for CABG instead of heparin for protamine allergic patients.

Hypercarbia limits PAO2 & therefore PaO2. Look at alveolar gas equation.

Hyperventilation (alkalosis) & hypothermia can decrease levels of ionized Calcium.

Hypothermia shifts CO2 response curve to right (like opiates) and can delay emergence.

Hypoxic ventilatory drive occurs usually when PO2 is below 50mmHg.

IgA is most likely cause of anaphylactic rxn in pt who has previously been transfused.

Low MAC of VAs has > effect on ventilatory response to hypoxemia than to hypercapnia.

Mendelson's Syndrome – gastric aspiration, hypoxemia, pulm edema, pulm HTN, dec'd pulm compliance.

Metoclopramide contraindicated in pheo -> can cause release of catecholamines.

Nitrous (50%) does NOT shift the CO_2 response curve.

Omeprazole (PPI) not reliable as H2 blockers. Decr dose in liver dz. Can cause myalgias, angioedema, & anaphylaxis.

Patients serum has no factors (but has antibodies, etc) Plasma has factors (no RBCs or platelets).

Platelet (6pack/1unit) has same level of factors as 1 unit of FFP.

Platelet life 10 days, RBC life 120 days.

PTT screens for levels of 5&8. If >1.5x normal then give FFP.

Repiratory quotient (CO_2/O_2) normal is 0.8. 200mL of CO_2 are produced for every 250mL O_2 used (0.8).

Starting doses: SNP 1mcg/kg/min, NTG 1mcg/kg/min, Epi 0.01mcg/kg/min

Test for hemolytic transfusion rxn is free Hb with Direct coombs test.

Transexamic acid & aminocaproic acid (Amicar) protect clot. Urokinase & TPA eat clot.

V/Q mismatch = Incr'd Aa gradient; Diffusion impairment = R-> L intracardiac shunt

WRT ventilatory control central (brainstem) modulate in response to pH and $PaCO_2$ (much faster/sensitive).

WRT ventilatory control peripheral (carotid/aortic receptors) modulate in response to arterial hypoxemia.

2010 ASRA Neuraxial & Regional Anticoagulation Guidelines Condensed

Heparin (activates anti-thrombin III -> inhibits IIa, Xa, and others)

> SQ (mini-dose) – No contraindication to neuraxial techniques unless pt has been receiving for >4 days –> then need only to obtain plt count (prior to placement or before removal of indwelling catheter) for risk of HIT.
>
> IV (dosing) – If required for vascular surg, etc then heparin dose should be delayed one hour after needle placement. Need to wait 2-4 hrs after last dose before removing indwelling catheter. Wait for re-heparinizaiton 2 hrs after catheter removal. Monitor post op with frequent motor checks.
>
> For Bloody tap – no evidence to support canceling case; discuss with surgeon.
>
> NB – For high risk pts, post-op monitoring of neurologic fxn & choosing neuraxial solutions that minimize motor blockade is recommended. Caution if other anticoagulants being administered (ASA, NSAIDS, etc).

LMWH (activates anti-thrombin III -> inhibits mainly factor Xa, peak @ 2 hrs, prolonged in renal dz)

> Pre-op – wait 10-12 hrs after last dose; If high dose (eg 1mg/kg BID) wait 24 hrs.
>
> For Bloody tap – delay LMWH until 24 hrs post-op.
>
> Single Day dosing – Give 1st dose 6-8 hrs post-op, & 2nd dose no sooner than 24 hrs after 1st dose. Indwelling catheters may be maintained. Wait 10-12 hrs after last dose prior to removal of catheter and wait at least 2 hrs after removal for subsequent dose.
>
> BID dosing – Give no earlier than 24 hrs post-op & 1st dose @ least 2 hrs after catheter removal. Do NOT leave catheter in place during therapeutic dosing such as this. Epidural catheter can be left in place overnight but removed 2 hrs prior to 1st dose as above.
>
> NB – no evidence that anti-Xa level is predictive of bleeding risk. Don't order it.

Warfarin (inhibits vit k dependent synthesis of factors 2/7/9/10; mostly 7, therapeutic INR 2-3)

> Pre-op Chronic use – Ideally intake should be stopped 4-5 days prior to procedure & PT/INR measured (<1.5 = WNL) prior to initiation of neuraxial block. Caution if other anticoagulants being administered (ASA, NSAIDS, Plavix, Heparin, LMWH, etc).
>
> Pre-op Initation – PT/INR should be checked if 1st dose was >24 hrs earlier, or if 2nd dose has been given.
>
> Re-initiation – neuraxial catheters should be removed (likely the AM of next day) when INR is <1.5 (corresponds to clotting factor activity levels of > 40%).
>
> NB – PT/INR should be monitored on daily basis. If INR >3 should prompt physician to lower dose in pts with indwelling catheters. Frequent neurologic testing (sensory/motor) should be employed 24 hrs after removal of catheter. Timing is somewhat tricky with Warfarin.

Antiplatelet Medications (diverse effects on platelet function)

> NSAIDS/ASA – alone do not increase risk of spinal hematoma. Caution if combo with above.
>
> Clopidogrel/Ticlodipine – discontinue 7 & 14 days prior to neuraxial technique respectively.
>
> GP IIb/IIIa inhibitors (octreotide) – contraindicated within 4 wks of surgery, await plt fxn recovery

Herbals: Garlic (inhibits platelet aggregation), Ginseng (inhibits platelet activating factor), & Ginko (↑ s PT). No evidence for mandatory cessation, caution w/combos.

Newer Anticoagulants: Fondiparinux (Xa inhibitor) & Thombin inhibitors (Argatroban, Lepirudin, etc) Advise against neuraxial techniques.

Deep Plexus & Peripheral Nerve Blocks: new advisory is to follow same recommendations to avoid severe hematoma. Excessive bleeding is more of concern than neurologic injury. Unclear if ultrasound techniques Δ morbidity.

This list is concise, not comprehensive. The main goal is to reduce the incidence of spinal hematoma. As always, each case should be looked at from an individual basis with clinical perspective. For further reference see ASRA website.

References
(in decreasing order of utilization)

1. Miller, Ronald, et al. Miller's Anesthesia. Churchill Livingstone, 7th Ed. 2009. Print

2. Hall, BA & Chantigian, RC. Anesthesia: A Comprehensive Review. Mosby, 4th Ed. 2010. Print

3. Barash, Paul. Clinical Anesthesia. Lippincott Williams & Wilkins, 6th Ed. 2009. Print

4. Marino, Paul. The ICU book, Lippincott Williams & Wilkins, 3rd Ed. 2006. Print

5. Litman, Ronald. Pediatric Anesthesia: The Requisites, Mosby, 1st Ed. 2004. Print

6. Leung, Jacqueline. Cardiac and Vascular Anesthesia: The Requisites, Mosby, 1st Ed. 2004. Print

7. Jensen, Niels. Big Blue: Anesthesiology Board Review Course Material, 2008. Print

8. Euliano, T. & Gravenstein, J. Essential Anesthesia: From Science to Practice. Cambridge University Press, 2nd Ed. 2011. Print

9. Horlocker, Terese T. MD; Wedel, Denise J. MD. 2010 January/February. Anticoagulation 3rd Edition. Regional Anesthesia and Pain Medicine:Volume 35, Issue 1, pp 64-101. ASRA Practice Advisory

Made in the USA
Lexington, KY
16 May 2015